OPIOIDS: ADDICTION, NARRATIVE, FREEDOM

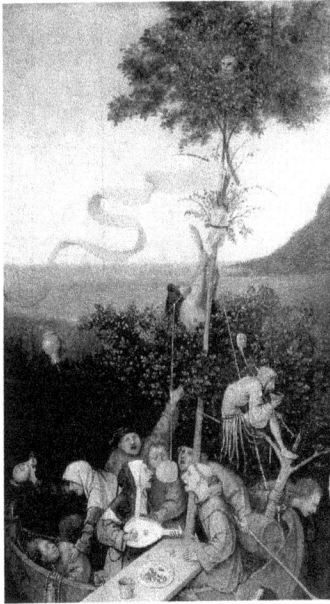

Fig. 1. Hieronymus Bosch, Ship of Fools (1490–1500)

Opioids

Addiction ◦ Narrative ◦ Freedom

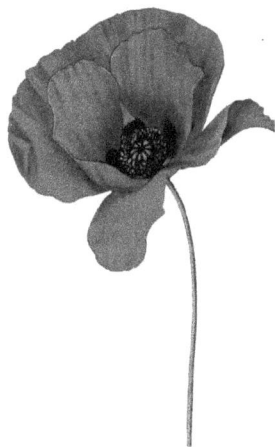

Maia Dolphin-Krute

Brainstorm Books
Santa Barbara, California

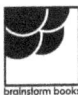

brainstorm books

First published in 2018 by Brainstorm Books
An imprint of punctum books, Earth, Milky Way
www.punctumbooks.com

ISBN-13: 978-1-947447-83-7 (print)
ISBN-13: 978-1-947447-84-4 (ePDF)

LCCN: 2018957173
Library of Congress Cataloging Data is available from the Library of Congress

Editorial team: Hannah Carlson, Jamilla Feemster, Kristen McCants, and Isaac Mikulski
Book design: Hannah Carlson, Kristen McCants, and Isaac Mikulski
Cover design: Hannah Carlson and Vincent W.J. van Gerven Oei

Contents

Acknowledgments

In many hopefully obvious ways, this book is dedicated to those who have died in relation to opioids during the timeframe of this writing, 2016–2018.

In addition to this dedication, I would like to thank all of the people who have talked with me and shared their experiences with and around opioids and pain (as well as those I simply think of often), in no particular order: Valerie, Pete, Lauren, Patrick, David, Max, Magali, Michael, Nancy, Julie, Meghann, PJ, Tony, Sean, Dan. In particular, my ongoing conversation and collaboration with Jesse Erin Posner is something I will always be thankful for.

As always, none of this would have been possible without the support of Eileen Joy at punctum books and the wonderful team at the Brainstorm Books imprint. I have been so happy to continue our working relationship and feel privileged to be included in the work punctum books does.

Everyday, I am grateful for the Dolphins, the Krutes, and the Dolphin-Krutes, for Dr. Peter Banks and Dr. Mohammed Issa, and especially for Jesse Kenas Collins.

The Opioid Epidemic: 2018

I am a pain patient. I am a patient being treated for pain as part of a chronic illness. Given contemporary medical technology and knowledge, this means that I am treated with a class of prescription drugs called opioids, or opioid painkillers. Because my pain is daily, my proximity to these substances is daily as well. This dailyness is constituted temporally in that they exist as an always possible physical experience and encounter, and one that has become synonymous with pain, now, and the thing larger than it: relief. Physically, my proximity becomes daily inasmuch as I am sitting three feet away from two different kinds of opioids right now, as usual, with a prescription for a third kind in my name, a few states away and unfilled. It was too strong for me.

In slightly farther distance from my body yet remaining in definite proximity are multiple other sites of opioids, places where they have become concentrated, in and around where I live in Boston. "Methadone Mile" is a common name for one such place, a stretch of streets surrounding several medical centers which have become some of the only drug abuse treatment sites nearby.[1] People concentrate there; I am about forty minutes

1   Nestor Ramos and Evan Alan, "Life and Loss on Methadone Mile,"

away. Closer still is Harvard Square, an area long known for its resident homeless and itinerant population, and it is this population I often wonder about when moving through the area on a weekly basis: which people are in even closer proximity to me than I can tell?

We are in proximity because this is the opioid epidemic.

"Opioid epidemic" names a present historical and historic moment centered on the substance of opioids, the number of people currently using and/or abusing them, and the number of people dying as a result of their repeated exposure and deep proximity to opioids. As of the most recent statistics, approximately 33,000 people are dying of opioid overdoses in America every year; this number includes both prescription drug overdoses and those from heroin and other illegal opioids.[2] This number is especially important as an overview because it emphasizes mass: "epidemic" names a quantity (a large quantity of bodies) situated temporally (for the past twenty-five years, all of the bodies abusing opioids at the same time) and geographically (in the same place; in the US, with regional foci taking on additional importance) and the quality this relationship produces — a crisis.

Moving towards or away from "Methadone Mile," from Harvard Square, from the Northeast generally and ultimately the US itself, I am never not in proximity to this crisis, its qualities and quantities. Particularly as a pain patient, I am never not entangled. No one is truly apart from this: opioids also exist as a set of endogenous biochemicals, a group of chemicals called endorphins that are produced by all humans and many other animals. Every human body is within this mass.

Tracing these proximities and entanglements around, within, and between bodies thus takes on an ethical urgency. Many of the terms at stake here ("freedom," "liberty," "pain," "willpower") have come to be figured as so deeply paradoxical within postmodern critique and culture as to seem, at the least, staid, and at the worst, empty. But within the same day of your having

The Boston Globe, July 2016, https://apps.bostonglobe.com/graphics/2016/07/methadone-mile/.

2 Centers for Disease Control and Prevention (CDC), "Opioid Overdose," October 23, 2017, https://www.cdc.gov/drugoverdose/.

read this, 152 people will have died of an opioid overdose. When I began writing, it was 97 people everyday. These deaths are urgent, and re-imbue such terms with the weight of an urgency in relation to a mass of bodies.

In beginning this way, with the statement that I am a pain patient, I mean to both disclose, up front, my privileged (if paradoxically so; I am, after all, in pain most of the time) position within the social, legal, and medical parameters of the opioid epidemic, as well as to outline the form and function of this text as an autoethnography, and one of a field I cannot help but be involved in. In methodology, this autoethnography is at once slightly off and perfectly suited to its contemporary crisis-time. It is an autoethnography at a slight remove: I look around. I sense proximities. It is a study of this act of looking around, a study of distances between bodies, a study of "the news," a study of science journalism, the pharmaceutical industry, and the government. There are no interviews, participants, case studies, or otherwise in-person material collected through standard anthropological methods. I stay where I am. Where I am, though, is frequently described as one of the epicenters of the epidemic. My neighbors, my friends, my coworkers: everyone has been affected in one way or another. Everyone I know knows someone who has overdosed, died, or otherwise takes or has taken opioids. At the same time, it is an autoethnography from the deepest point of immersion and involvement possible by being dependent on and attending to what is (going on) biologically and pharmaceutically in my body.

Because of the specifics of my body and its position in relation to opioids, I am a pain patient; in opposing relation to the specifics named "pain patient," other people become "junkies" or similar terms. These people are not who I am writing about; or, I am not writing about people within these terms. These terms portray the epidemic to be somehow one-dimensional, as if this was not also about the very real and equally life-threatening negativity of the systemic violence currently contributing to the proliferation of bodies and lives within the zone of addiction. At the same time, I see the people who are dying. And I recognize the life-threatening nature of the actions and triggers called "addiction" as being rooted within biological and neurological human systems. In short, I understand addiction as a relapsing and remitting brain disease. I do not think people can "just stop" any more than they "just" started; I offer zero moral judgment. I understand this as chronic, despite the presumed and imposed temporal bounds set by the idea of an epidemic. Through its chronicity, addiction becomes entangled with the historical, with a history of capitalism and the development of biopolitical institutions and their aims. In looking around, this is one set of proximities I seek to feel out: why now? What is the relationship between a historical and historic moment, present moments, moments within capitalism, and a set of repeated neurological activities, human desire, and loss that has fueled the exponential rise in the rates of opioid use and abuse between 2000–2016? I look towards epidemiology and the study of bodily statistics as well as mass media narratives that seek to answer this question; these narratives and statistics are the focus of the first chapter. I am not interested in whether such narratives are right or wrong, but more interested in why it's these explanations that are being given and how the beliefs underlying them can come to be understood as, ultimately, expressions of a contemporary affective structure or its dismantling. What does it feel like to be within the opioid epidemic? What is the structure, the scaffolding or support, of an experiential encounter amid precarity, loss, economics, racism, and painkillers?

In feeling out how the opioid epidemic is taking shape affectively, I turn in the second chapter to examine what addiction itself feels like. As with any chronic disease, addiction is deeply formed by temporal cycles and patterns, from the narrative arc named by "relapsing and remitting" to the routine of getting high, coming down. While there exists an entire genre of memoir dedicated to addiction narratives, a genre that rapidly proliferated throughout the 1990s and 2000s and is exemplified by books like *Night of the Gun* and *Another Bullshit Night in Suck City,* these memoirs are generally dedicated to telling an overall story of a (finished and recovered from) addiction, always reliant on autobiographical interest and ultimate redemption. What becomes more valuable and telling within the context of the opioid epidemic are not the larger personal and completed stories, but the minutiae of a daily and ongoing addiction.

In delineating a taxonomy of time within addiction, even one that can only ever remain partial, having been written from the perspective of someone not living within their own addiction, we can come into a zone of encounter between opioids, those who use them, and government. How are the bounds of "pain patient" and "junkie" being set by the assumed temporal qualities of the bodies involved? How are determinations about time producing kinds of citizens? What forms of citizenship are possible within the opioid epidemic when in deep proximity to these substances?

Embedded in and motivating a set of behaviors within addiction as a chronic disease are a set of neurological activities and relationships set to and setting an additional kind of time. Opioids, both those that enter a body from the outside as well as those found endogenously within it, play a key role in multiple neurological processes dealing with the sensation of physical pain and a bodily reaction to it: for instance, endorphins play a key role in placebo responses, to which I turn in the final chapter. As will be explored in detail, a placebo pain-relieving response is a function of social relationships and expectations about time, and the time one's body is about to be in. By thinking through and with that "about to be," in combination with ideas of a Marxist *freedom with,* ideas of freedom as a relational and contextual practice (as formulated in the writing of Jean-Luc Nancy and others), how can we envision what happens near the end or after an epidemic of these proportions, whose foundations rest on ideas of what it means to be a citizen within a historically-specific material environment set against social and economic factors? Or, how do you live with something for a long time? What forms of freedom become possible when continually modulated by physical experience and proximity to substances? How can we maintain or exit from our proximities?

In the intervening chapters, I focus on two main aspects of or towards these final questions. In chapter three, I examine the materiality of opioids, their standing as substances throughout economic history and what, exactly, there is to be in proximity to. How has it happened that the current environment has become so deeply saturated by opioids that 41% of Americans report knowing someone who has abused these drugs?[3] It is and is not really the first time something like this has happened. On the one hand, there is a long history of building risk into an environment, quite literally. From asbestos to lead, we have always lived in an environment awash with risky materials. On the other hand, the parameters of mass involvement and the fact that opioids concurrently play a vital and beneficial role within medicine make the risks of now unique. In examining a relationship between material risks in a built environment and the laws that legislate and, sometimes, abate those risks, I ask questions about a hierarchy of risk, of exposure, and who determines which populations are and should be more or less exposed. The time of the opioid epidemic has also seen such material risk crises as the lead found in the water of Flint, MI, and the contaminated soil recently discovered around public housing in Indiana: such cases illuminate the systems of power through which substances move and are moved. Within this context, what can "substance abuse" mean and come to include?

Lastly, I turn to the most deeply autoethnographic proximity: the case of pain patients. Recently passed legislation in multiple states has seen ever-increasing regulation of prescription opioids, in an effort to curb an obvious flow of these substances, and to stem their movement from licit to illicit in standing. Responses to such regulations from governmental and medical bodies have been largely positive, lauding these efforts against the opioid epidemic. Pain patients, on the other hand, have expressed concern (seen in widely-published articles and op-eds) over a continuation of their ability to access what are also life-saving, quality-of-life-enhancing medications.[4] To complicate this

3 Dylan Scott, "1 in 3 Americans Blame Doctors for National Opioid Epidemic, STAT-Harvard Poll Finds," STAT, March 17, 2016, https://www.statnews.com/2016/03/17/stat-harvard-opioid-poll/.

4 See Bob Tedeschi, "A 'Civil War' Over Painkillers Rips Apart the Medical Community — and Leaves Patients in Fear," STAT, January 17, 2017, https://www.statnews.com/2017/01/17/chronic-pain-management-opioids/, and Stefan Kertesz and Sally Satel, "Some People Still Need Opioids," Slate, August 17, 2017, http://www.slate.com/articles/health_and_science/medical_examiner/2017/08/cutting_down_on_

binary of "good medicine" and "bad drugs" further, current data shows that it is not always true that lowering prescribing rates will also lower drug abuse: in Massachusetts, where prescribing rates and the number of opioid prescriptions have decreased in 2016, the number of overdose deaths throughout the state is on track to make 2017 the worst year yet.[5] While this case may make an obvious argument about causality and confusion, the conflict it demonstrates over how best to address the needs and pain of both pain patients and drug users points to deeper ideas and questions: how much of the opioid epidemic is constituted by what is and is not being called pain? How can this conflict within legislation and medical treatment demonstrate the very real categorization and hierarchizing of pain, as well as of the desires that become embedded and perpetuated within and in proximity to pain? Beyond affect, legislation, or medicine, much of the answers to these questions will be economic in nature. Pain represents billions of dollars. One opioid medication alone, OxyContin, has generated an estimated $35 billion in revenue since its release in the 1990s.[6] Pain is money, in so many forms and at so many points within the opioid epidemic and responses to it. The enormity of the money of pain should never not be seen in relation to the enormity of the opioid epidemic.

And how will this enormity come to pass? How do we envision what happens after an epidemic? Or, drawing on an understanding of "post-" to mean "in the middle of the crisis of," perhaps we can only ever be in a post-opioid period, an affective and political situation not necessarily dependent on drug use statistics alone; perhaps we are all already too enveloped.

opioids_has_made_life_miserable_for_chronic_pain_patients.html.

5 Martha Bebinger, "New Numbers Show Opioid Epidemic Rages on in Massachusetts," *CommonHealth* (blog), *WBUR,* August 3, 2016, http://www.wbur.org/commonhealth/2016/08/03/opioid-epidemic-numbers.

6 Alex Morell, "The OxyContin Clan: The $14 Billion Newcomer to Forbes 2015 List of Richest U.S. Families," *Forbes,* July 1, 2015, http://www.forbes.com/sites/alexmorrell/2015/07/01/the-oxycontin-clan-the-14-billion-newcomer-to-forbes-2015-list-of-richest-u-s-families/#14cb7821c0e2.

1

Narrative

The Opioid Epidemic

The opioid epidemic is what has happened, what is happening now, and what is about to happen to many people in proximity to a group of substances called opioids within the United States. Depending on how one defines the specifics of a proximity to opioids, and thus how many of which bodies should be counted, as well as the years that are determined to fall into what has happened, now, and next, the exact numbers for defining the scope of the opioid epidemic will vary. The opioid epidemic is 33,000 people dying of overdoses in 2015;[1] the opioid epidemic is 2.1 million Americans with substance abuse issues related to prescription drugs;[2] the opioid epidemic is the National Institute

[1] Centers for Disease Control and Prevention (CDC), "Opioid Overdose," October 23, 2017, https://www.cdc.gov/drugoverdose/.
[2] Nora D. Volkow, "America's Addiction to Opioids: Heroin and Prescription Drug Abuse," National Institute on Drug Abuse (NIDA), May 14, 2014, https://www.drugabuse.gov/about-nida/legislative-activities/testimony-to-congress/2018/americas-addiction-to-opioids-heroin-prescription-drug-abuse.

on Drug Abuse launching its first prescription drug abuse public health initiative in 2001;[3] the opioid epidemic is a 50% increase in fatal heroin overdoses between the early 2000s and 2010;[4] the opioid epidemic is a 73% increase in synthetic opioid-related deaths in 2015;[5] the opioid epidemic is just over 10,000 overdoses involving heroin in 2014;[6] the opioid epidemic is 80% of heroin users first starting to abuse opioids through prescription medications;[7] the opioid epidemic is 91 people dying of opioid overdoses every day;[8] the opioid epidemic is the fact that now, several months after first writing this sentence, the opioid epidemic is 142 people dying of opioid overdoses every day;[9] the opioid epidemic is 1,000 people receiving emergency treatment for opioid-related injuries daily;[10] the opioid epidemic is a 500% increase in neonatal abstinence syndrome between 2000–2012;[11] the opioid epidemic is 90% of heroin users being white, on average 23 years old, and more likely to live in rural or suburban

3 Volkow, "America's Addiction to Opioids."

4 Volkow, "America's Addiction to Opioids."

5 Rose A. Rudd, Puja Seth, Felicita David, and Lawrence Scholl, "Increases in Drug and Opioid-Involved Overdose Deaths–United States, 2010–2015," *Morbidity and Mortality Weekly Report,* CDC, December 30, 2016, https://www.cdc.gov/mmwr/volumes/65/wr/mm655051e1.htm.

6 Volkow, "What Science Tells Us About Opioid Abuse and Addiction," NIDA, January 27, 2016, https://www.drugabuse.gov/about-nida/legislative-activities/testimony-to-congress/2018/what-science-tells-us-about-opioid-abuse-addiction.

7 Theodore J. Cicero, Matthew S. Ellis, Hilary L. Surratt, et al., "The Changing Face of Heroin Use in the United States: A Retrospective Analysis of the Past 50 Years," *JAMA Psychiatry* 71, no. 7 (July 2014): 821–26, https://doi.org/10.1001/jamapsychiatry.2014.366.

8 CDC, "Understanding the Epidemic," August 30, 2017, https://www.cdc.gov/drugoverdose/epidemic/index.html.

9 Grace Donnelly, "As Drug Overdoses Hit Record High, Trump Offers Little on Opioid Policy," *Fortune,* August 8, 2017, http://fortune.com/2017/08/08/record-high-drug-related-death-rate-2016/.

10 Harvard T.H. Chan School of Public Health, "An Opioid Emergency," November 2, 2017, https://www.hsph.harvard.edu/news/multimedia-article/president-trump-opioid-emergency/.

11 Volkow, "What Science Tells Us About Opioid Abuse and Addiction."

settings rather than urban ones;[12] the opioid epidemic is 174 over-doses in a single six-day span in Ohio;[13] the opioid epidemic is the estimated sales of OxyContin at $35 billion since its release in 1995;[14] the opioid epidemic is 41% of Americans who say they know someone who has abused prescription drugs;[15] the opioid epidemic is opioid overdoses killing more people than heroin and cocaine combined;[16] the opioid epidemic is hydrocodone (i.e. Vicodin) products being the most prescribed drug in the United States and the second most abused prescription opioid;[17] the opioid epidemic is the $880 billion spent on lobbying efforts by opioid drug manufacturers, an amount eight times that spent by the gun lobby for the same period;[18] the opioid epidemic is the 2.1 million people who misused prescription opioids for the first time and the 948,000 people who used heroin during 2016;[19] the

12 Cicero, et al., "The Changing Face of Heroin Use in the United States."
13 Katie Mettler, "'This is unprecedented': 174 Heroin Overdoses in 6 Days in Cincinnati," *Chicago Tribune,* August 29, 2016, http://www.chicagotribune.com/news/nationworld/midwest/ct-heroin-overdose-outbreak-20160829-story.html.
14 Alex Morell, "The OxyContin Clan: The $14 Billion Newcomer to Forbes 2015 List of Richest U.S. Families," *Forbes,* July 1, 2015, http://www.forbes.com/sites/alexmorrell/2015/07/01/the-oxycontin-clan-the-14-billion-newcomer-to-forbes-2015-list-of-richest-u-s-families/#14cb7821c0e2.
15 Dylan Scott, "1 in 3 Americans Blame Doctors for National Opioid Epidemic, STAT-Harvard Poll Finds," *STAT,* March 17, 2017, https://www.statnews.com/2016/03/17/stat-harvard-opioid-poll/.
16 Jerome Schofferman, Scott M. Fishman, and R. Norman Harden, "Did We Reach Too Far? The Opioid Epidemic and Chronic Pain," *American Academy of Physical Medicine and Rehabilitation* 6, no. 1 (January 2014): 78–84, https://doi.org/10.1016/j.pmrj.2013.12.003.
17 Schofferman, "There is a Role for Long-term Opioid Analgesics in Well-selected Patients With Chronic, Severe, and Refractory Spine Pain," in Schofferman, Fishman, and Harden, "Did We Reach Too Far?" 79–80.
18 Erin Brodwin, "A Searing New Report Claims Opioid Drugmakers Spent 8 times as Much as the NRA on Lobbying," *Business Insider,* September 19, 2016, http://www.businessinsider.com/new-ap-report-opioid-drugmakers-outspent-nra-lobbying-2016-9.
19 Health and Human Services (HHS), "The Opioid Epidemic: By the

opioid epidemic is drug overdoses being the leading cause of accidental death in the United States;[20] the opioid epidemic is the rise in suicide rates, particularly in rural areas, between 2000–2015;[21] the opioid epidemic is overdose deaths surpassing fatalities from both gun homicides and traffic accidents;[22] the opioid epidemic is how, in Massachusetts, opioid-related deaths have increased by 350% since 2000, and how these deaths represent more than a third of all deaths in people ages 25–34;[23] the opioid epidemic is 259 million prescriptions given for opioids in 2012;[24] the opioid epidemic is death rates related to opioids now rivaling those of AIDS during the 1990s;[25] the opioid epidemic is a 369% increase in opioid overdose deaths in 15 years (1999–2014);[26] the opioid epidemic is prescribing rates for opioids nearly tripling over 20 years;[27] the opioid epidemic is how 12 states have had more opioid prescriptions than people in recent years;[28] the opioid epidemic is how America represents 5 percent of the world's popula-

Numbers," updated January 2018, https://www.hhs.gov/opioids/sites/default/files/2018-01/opioids-infographic.pdf.

20 Katharine Q. Seelye, "As Drug Deaths Soar, a Silver Lining for Transplant Patients," *The New York Times,* October 6, 2016, https://www.nytimes.com/2016/10/06/us/as-drug-deaths-soar-a-silver-lining-for-organ-transplant-patients.html?ref=todayspaper&_r=0.

21 Joel Achenbach and Dan Keating, "A New Divide in American Death," *The Washington Post,* April 10, 2016, http://www.washingtonpost.com/sf/national/2016/04/10/a-new-divide-in-american-death/?utm_term=.3dbded6c06f5.

22 Seelye, "As Drug Deaths Soar, a Silver Lining for Transplant Patients."

23 Massachusetts Department of Public Health, "Data Brief: An Assessment of Opioid-Related Deaths in Massachusetts, 2013–2014," September 2016, https://www.mass.gov/files/documents/2016/09/pn/chapter-55-opioid-overdose-study-data-brief-9-15-2016.pdf.

24 American Society of Addiction Medicine, "Opioid Addiction: 2016 Facts & Figures," n.d., http://www.asam.org/docs/default-source/advocacy/opioid-addiction-disease-facts-figures.pdf.

25 Dan Nolan and Chris Amico, "How Bad is the Opioid Epidemic?" *PBS Frontline,* February 23, 2016, http://www.pbs.org/wgbh/frontline/article/how-bad-is-the-opioid-epidemic/.

26 Nolan and Amico, "How Bad is the Opioid Epidemic?"

27 Nolan and Amico, "How Bad is the Opioid Epidemic?"

28 Nolan and Amico, "How Bad is the Opioid Epidemic?"

tion but consumes 80 percent of its prescription opioids;[29] the opioid epidemic is 186,000 Americans dying from prescription drug overdoses since 2000;[30] the opioid epidemic is the 1 in 12 Americans who know someone who has died from a prescription drug overdose.[31]

The numbers are not in and of themselves descriptions. These numbers do not make clear the medical or legal status of the bodies they count. These numbers, especially those related to prescribing rates, do not distinguish between medications given in emergency settings, those given for long-term pain management, and those distributed by clinics referred to as "pill mills." Nor do the numbers alone give a clear idea of the temporal nature of the opioid epidemic, when it began or if it may have ended; though the statistics may seem to make apparent the timeframe (the 1990s through the 2000s, to today), all it is actually safe to assume about this is that this is the timeframe being examined and compared. In part, this lack of clarity is not confined to the numbers but reflects an overall lack of consensus (among governing public health groups and the media that interprets their findings) about the exact beginning of the opioid epidemic. The opioid epidemic began in the 1990s, with the release and mass promotion of new drugs like OxyContin that had little if any abuse-deterrents built into them and were themselves, in part, built on a denial of the abuse potential inherent in opioids; the opioid epidemic begin in 1995 when medical governing bodies proclaimed pain to be the fifth vital sign and, as such, in need of (aggressive) monitoring and treatment, contributing to the rise in opioid prescribing rates;[32] the opioid epidemic began in the mid-2000s as the recreational use of opioids began to rise rapidly and spread throughout economically depressed, post-industrial towns located primarily in the Ohio River Valley, the Appalachians, and the US Rust Belt; the opioid epidemic began

29 Achenbach and Keating, "A New Divide in American Death."
30 CDC, "Understanding the Epidemic."
31 Scott, "1 in 3 Americans Blame Doctors for National Opioid Epidemic."
32 Sam Quinones, *Dreamland: The True Tale of America's Opiate Epidemic* (London: Bloomsbury, 2015), 115.

when large numbers of white people began dying; the opioid epidemic began as Mexican and Columbian heroin production rose in an equally rapid manner in the mid-2000s;[33] the opioid epidemic began in 2014 when, for the first time, the number of opioid-related deaths surpassed those from traffic accidents.[34] The opioid epidemic is a leading cause of death.

I have gathered almost all of these statistics from articles that have appeared over the past two years in major news sources, most for a general audience, though some are specific to medical, healthcare, or science news; the rest of the numbers are gathered from government sources such as the Centers for Disease Control and Prevention (CDC), the Food and Drug Administration (FDA), the National Institutes of Health (NIH), and the National Institute for Drug Abuse (NIDA), in addition to state-level public health and health and human services departments. For now, I would like to focus on articles appearing in the news and their narratives; I will attend to the governmental sources later in this text, relative to the level of legal regulations and responses to the opioid epidemic. Such articles can roughly be divided into two main groups according to the type of narrative they exemplify. The first are articles which focus on an overarching narrative of the opioid epidemic and *why* it is happening. These narratives tend to look for one to two main causes and are set against a backdrop of pharmaceutical development, medical mismanagement, and economic recession, or they choose to focus on the demographics of the opioid epidemic itself. As if the kinds of people involved are what need explaining. The second set of articles forgoes an obviously overarching narrative to focus instead on the personal story of one person or a small group of people, generally people

---

33 NIDA, "Increased Drug Availability is Associated with Increased Use and Overdose," January 2018, https://www.drugabuse.gov/publications/research-reports/relationship-between-prescription-drug-abuse-heroin-use/increased-drug-availability-associated-increased-use-overdose.

34 For statistics on motor vehicle deaths and accidental poisoning deaths, 90% of which can be attributed to drug overdoses, see the CDC, "Accidents or Unintentional Injuries," March 17, 2017, http://www.cdc.gov/nchs/fastats/accidental-injury.htm.

who have either themselves "battled" opioid addiction or have lost an immediate loved one to an opioid-related death. While focusing on the personal, these articles do not entirely neglect a larger narrative arc and tend to function as microcosms for the recent history of a specific town or small region. The multiplicity of these narratives both in terms of sheer quantity of coverage as well as internal variety and variation in the causes described can be taken as representative of the urgency in needing to understand why now is happening, the number of points of view for doing so, and the dense entanglement of systems generating this situation. Stylistically, these articles span conventions taken from the human interest piece, the redemption narrative, and the addiction memoir to longform science journalism and investigative reporting, and do so by incorporating data journalism and popular neuroscience.

The causes detailed in both sets of narratives are representative of various combinations of statistics and timeframes: the opioid epidemic is a leading cause of death because of doctors who have recklessly over-prescribed opioid medications since the 1990s; the opioid epidemic is a leading cause of death because of people who are irresponsible when it comes to what they're putting into their bodies, though they can most often not be faulted for this, living as they do in economically depressed towns with high rates of unemployment which are concurrently flooded with incoming heroin from Mexico, opioids distributed through "pill mills" (clinics run by a specific subset of aforementioned reckless doctors), or both; the opioid epidemic is a leading cause of death because of doctors who are over-prescribing to "everyday people," taken to mean both white people and people who would otherwise simply be recovering from an ordinary injury or surgery, but whose recovery was interrupted by the sheer addictiveness of the drugs they were given;[35] the opioid epidemic is a leading cause of death. Perhaps part of the confusion in identifying a single and clear cause of the epidemic is surprise at

35 Maura Healy, "Cutting Off the Opioid Epidemic at the Root," *The Boston Globe,* February 16, 2016, https://www.bostonglobe. com/opinion/2016/02/16/cutting-off-opioid-epidemic-root/ EdovYeSsn5QbWtLY3ICY5J/story.html.

the paradox of its having happened within this timeframe. That is, beginning in the 1990s or early 2000s, the opioid epidemic is taking place in the immediate wake of the War on Drugs, initiated in the 1970s and having been redoubled through the 1990s. In 1999, the US Office of National Drug Control Policy released its *National Drug Control Strategy,* a report that detailed efforts focused almost entirely on reducing the global supply of illicit substances, with the aim of achieving "the lowest recorded drug use rate in American history."[36]

Leading causes of death are, understandably, often subject to this kind of explanatory narrativizing and collective imagining. Or bargaining. A stark example can be gathered from the media, both mass media and the official narratives and images distributed by the US government, in a post-WWII, Cold War-era psychological climate. The recent destruction of Hiroshima and Nagasaki, at that moment, was envisioned as "mass death perpetrated by industrial technologies,"[37] epitomized in the image of the mushroom cloud. Now, this is mass death perpetrated by pharmaceutical technologies, mass death perpetrated by dissolving racialized class structures, mass death perpetrated by dissolving desires predicated on the perpetuation of said class structures, mass death perpetrated by pain; ultimately, mass death perpetrated by mass death, epitomized in the image of the syringe.

The proliferation of this coverage and its convergence into these easily identifiable and so frequently repeated narratives is evidence of an emerging genre: opioid epidemic coverage. While referring to a form of journalism, "opioid epidemic coverage" should be read more as a descriptor of the narratives themselves, allowing for the way these narratives may, in the coming years, extend beyond ongoing coverage and take the form of opioid addiction memoirs, for instance. Taking genre to mean "a locus of affective situations that not only generate exemplary aesthetic

36 Alfred McCoy, "From Free Trade to Prohibition: A Critical History of the Modern Asian Opium Trade," *Fordham Urban Law Journal* 28, no. 1 (2000): 307–49, https://ir.lawnet.fordham.edu/ulj/vol28/iss1/4.

37 Alan Meek, *Biopolitical Media: Catastrophe, Immunity, and Bare Life* (New York: Routledge, 2016), 112.

conventions but exemplify political and subjective formations local to a particular time and space,"[38] I mean to deeply include (or implicate) opioid epidemic coverage as a genre and its specific affective, political, and subjective formations when I say "the opioid epidemic." The opioid epidemic is what is constructed around the opioid epidemic.

The opioid epidemic is what is constructed around the opioid epidemic because this is not the flu. It is not the influenza of 1912, nor is it measles, mumps, cholera, polio, typhoid, or tuberculosis. While to one degree or another it is true that each of these diseases and their epidemics were generative of their own affective and political situations, expressed primarily as judgments and moral valuations of the people involved, it is also true that none are entirely like the opioid epidemic. AIDS comes close, given the predominance of moralizing in coverage of those affected, and for this reason it is striking, in a PBS Frontline article, to see death rates from AIDS compared to those of the opioid epidemic;[39] though diseases, as Susan Sontag made famous, are always subject to becoming metaphors for kinds of people, it is rare to find an example of an epidemic and disease so clearly about kinds of people; *epidemics of people*. A crisis-time of proliferation, whether of the bodies of (dying, ignored) gay men or those of "junkies," a term which also names the dying and (deserving to be) ignored.

At the same time, the nature of the proliferation of "kinds of people" within the context of the opioid epidemic is paradoxical. It seems not that there are too many of a particular type of person within the United States — thus it seems that drug addicts themselves are not the fear — but that the kind of person proliferating within a zone of addiction and abuse is not the right kind. What opioid epidemic coverage makes clear in its attention to the demographics of those involved, whether explicitly or implicitly, is that *these are not the people who are supposed to be dying.* White people are not junkies, and they are not heroin addicts; "drug abuse" refers, in a deeply embedded

38 Lauren Berlant, *Cruel Optimism* (Durham, NC: Duke University Press, 2011), 66.
39 Nolan and Amico, "How Bad is the Opioid Epidemic?"

way, to a situation occupying inner city zones lived in entirely by minority populations. If mass media attention is paid to white drug abuse, it has almost always been in the form of sensationalizing suburban teenage drug trends (thus situating white drug abuse as a temporary phase that people grow out of) or bestselling memoirs written post-recovery (reinforcing the temporariness and ultimately individual triumph that can (only) be associated with white drug abuse). If this were not the belief, why would this coverage be necessary? If it were not believed that these are not the people who are supposed to be dying, why would explanations proliferate as to why it is *these* people and not others? If the opioid epidemic were contained to young minority men living in urban areas (which, historically, heroin use has been),[40] would this genre have emerged? Writing on the Cold War period, to continue our example, Joseph Masco noted that at that time "it became a civic obligation to imagine…the physical destruction of the nation state." This obligation was expressed not only through mass and governmental media but also in "civil defense simulation, evacuations, and drills," which came to constitute a "community under constant threat," one that Masco argues was an ultimately psychological maneuver to justify what were authoritarian regimes of surveillance and media control.[41] The emergence of the genre of opioid epidemic coverage demonstrates an ongoing civic obligation to imagine the physical destruction of the nation state through the destruction of one of its most privileged classes of people. Or what has seemed like its most privileged class; the obligation is to explain both the destruction and a contemporary affect dominated by a loss of privilege, a dissolve of "fantasies of the good life," and a concurrent loss of optimism.

In describing the opioid epidemic throughout this text and moving through, sitting in, dissolving into various proximities within it and alongside it, how will it be possible to avoid generic explanations while simultaneously being wary of impulses to instead find out "what is really going on"? This *is* what is really going on. At the same time, the opioid epidemic is not a mono-

40 Cicero, et al., "The Changing Face of Heroin Use in the United States."
41 Joseph Masco, quoted in Meek, *Biopolitical Media,* 118.

lithic event that can or should function as a cipher for ongoing, multifaceted social and economic situations that are indeed being expressed through the opioid epidemic and its genre, but also simultaneously through other social movements and political events (from #BlackLivesMatter to the rise of Donald Trump). The opioid epidemic does not explain everything, and attempting to use it as a construction for doing so is unethical, given how many people are dying, although doing so would not be without historical precedent; disasters, like illnesses, are also always subject to becoming metaphors. I will try to be in proximity to all of these explanatory forces, their paradoxes, and their metaphors.

Opioid epidemic coverage thus constitutes an affective situation predominated by feelings of disbelief and surprise, confusion, that are representative of a current political situation of ongoing racialized violence set in the context of a decade-long economic recession, mass unemployment, and other political economic changes. It is this convergence of affect, politics, and death as well as the narratives that actively seek to construct, dramatically and historically, the parameters of this convergence that I understand to be *the opioid epidemic,* and the dense configuration to which I mean to refer in using this term throughout.

White

In the 1960s, 82.8% of heroin users were young men, on average about 16 years old, whose first opioid used was heroin (as opposed to a prescription painkiller). In 2014, 90% of heroin users were white people, split more or less evenly by gender, who were more likely to live in less urban areas. On average, these recent opioid users are about 23 years old, and far more likely to have started using heroin after first using a prescription painkiller.[42] The opioid epidemic is young white people in rural areas abusing prescription drugs before beginning to use heroin. The opioid epidemic isn't what it used to be.

In part to avoid taking this set of demographic statistics as a totalizing image, I aim to examine what seem to be the three main components (white, 23 years old, rural) separately, though

42 Cicero, et al., "The Changing Face of Heroin Use in the United States."

also attending to their ongoing proximities. How can the whiteness of the opioid epidemic be set within a historical context that also takes into account the specificities of the current moment it is being actualized within? It is true that these recent demographics represent a shift from historical patterns of drug use, and this shift is significant in more ways than one. On a surface level, the shift represents apparent changes in patterns of use and the distribution of illicit substances; on this level, the shift is representative of a drug abuse epidemic conceptualized as a problem of too much of a substance in a particular time and place. On a deeper level is the paradigmatic break this shift represents. Historically, as in the young, urban, and male heroin users of the 1960s, there has always been a "connection of drug use with groups regarded as potentially dangerous or deviant."[43] Sitting within this broken connection, in proximity to the young white opioid users of recent years, is a representation of a drug abuse epidemic conceptualized as a problem of too much of a *kind of person* in a particular time and place; too much of a surprising kind of person; too much of a white person abusing drugs. The opioid epidemic isn't what it was.

It is also possible to contextualize the whiteness of the opioid epidemic without tracing all the way back to the 1960s; more recent history, going back to what is most frequently designated as the beginning of the opioid epidemic, the 1990s, is also deeply illuminating and explanatory. For example, within this timeframe, racial discrimination has been built into legal and medical practices related to opioids in such ways that would help to explain this whiteness. And by "help explain this whiteness," I mean contextualize this facet of the opioid epidemic such that it makes sense as a product of recent social histories and does not contribute to a feeling of it needing to be explained; this did not "just happen," nor did it happen in a sudden, surprising way, though this is not the same as saying that it could have been entirely predicted.

---

43 Alex Mold, "Consuming Habits: Histories of Drugs in Modern Societies," *Culture and Social History* 4, no. 2 (2007): 261–70, at 268, https://doi.org/10.2752/147800307X199074.

Legally, drug enforcement agencies (namely the DEA but also local and regional police forces) have focused their efforts on people of color throughout this time period. This period is the War on Drugs. "Of cases concluded in federal district courts since 1989, drug and public order cases…have increased at the greatest rate."[44] The length of prison sentences issued in drug cases has also increased, and currently stands at, on average, 59.7 months. Although surveys have found that 14 million whites and 2.6 million African Americans report using an illicit drug (approximately 5 times as many whites as African Americans), African Americans are sent to prison for drug offenses at a rate about 10 times that of whites. The amount of time an African American person spends in a prison sentence for a drug related abuse is virtually the same as the length served by a white person for a violent offense — close to 60 months.[45]

Compounding this is research that demonstrates clear racial bias in the distribution of pain medications in medical settings. A 2012 analysis of 20 years of published research found that African Americans are 34% less likely to be prescribed opioids than whites, in both acute and long-term situations.[46] Furthermore, African American patients are more likely to be referred for drug abuse assessments (such as increased urine drug testing) and less likely to be referred to a pain management specialist.[47] These discrepancies are continued in broader settings. Even in neighborhoods of similar income brackets, pharmacies in predominantly African American neighborhoods are less likely to stock opioids than pharmacies in mostly white areas; pharmacies in white

44 Bureau of Justice Statistics, "Drugs and Crime Facts: Pretrial, Prosecution, and Adjudication," n.d., https://www.bjs.gov/content/dcf/ptrpa.cfm.

45 NAACP, "Criminal Justice Fact Sheet," n.d., http://www.naacp.org/pages/criminal-justice-fact-sheet.

46 Abby Goodnough, "Finding Good Pain Treatment is Hard. If You're Not White, It's Even Harder," *The New York Times,* August 9, 2016, http://www.nytimes.com/2016/08/10/us/how-race-plays-a-role-in-patients-pain-treatment.html.

47 National Institutes of Health Pain Consortium, "Disparities in Pain Care," n.d., https://www.ninds.nih.gov/sites/default/files/DisparitiesPainCare.pdf.

neighborhoods are 54% more likely to stock opioids than those in African American ones.[48]

Taking these legal and medical discriminatory practices together, a clear picture emerges of a population — white people — that has been largely absent from drug enforcement practices while at the same time maintaining easy access to quantities of prescription drugs. Given that almost 80% of people involved in the opioid epidemic report first using a prescription opioid (instead of heroin), this access is an obvious vector for drug abuse and the distribution of opioids, or, at the least, representative of an initial point of entry into a proximity to this substance. Simultaneously, and counterintuitively, this vector is not as explanatory or perhaps as relevant, now, as it may once have been. The most recent statistics available for Massachusetts demonstrate a decline in prescribing rates of opioids, but overdose deaths related to opioids have only continued to increase; the epidemic is shifting.[49] At the same time, and perhaps to counter an explanatory impulse, contextualizing whiteness in this way does not explain whiteness; it demonstrates a possible cause as to why this population would be more effected, now, by opioids than other populations, but fails to account for the overwhelming surprise and confusion that ultimately surround not the large numbers of white people making up the opioid epidemic, but *the qualities of whiteness* the epidemic has become associated with. At the heart of explanations for the rise of opioid abuse among white people are not feelings towards an epidemiological cause, but feelings towards an explanation of a loss of privilege and the dissolution of known, entrenched (and therefore seemingly stable) class and social categories. The demographic explanations of opioid epidemic coverage thus, in a sense, seek not to explain the opioid epidemic but the construction of the opioid epidemic: how should the surrounding affective and political situation of the opioid epidemic, that seems to be directly

---

48 Goodnough, "Finding Good Pain Treatment is Hard."
49 Martha Bebinger, "New Numbers Show Opioid Epidemic Rages On in Massachusetts," *CommonHealth* (blog), *WBUR,* August 3, 2016, http://www.wbur.org/commonhealth/2016/08/03/opioid-epidemic-numbers.

contributing to our experience of it, be explained? How can we explain the loss(es) overlaying the deaths?

Expressions surrounding the whiteness of the opioid epidemic demonstrate a known/unknown and invisible/hypervisible duality that surrounds the bodies of those involved. This duality is exemplified in the generic rhetorical move of contextualizing opioids in the bodies of famous people: for example, "fentanyl, the prescription painkiller that led to the death earlier this year of the pop star Prince;"[50] "It was fentanyl…It's what killed the musician Prince;"[51] "Pop-music legend Prince died of an opioid fentanyl overdose in the spring, raising the visibility of the issue."[52] Such a move performs an implicit explanation that maintains a sense of the known-hypervisible by demonstrating through the very celebrity and quality of being a public figure how the event of an opioid overdose (and opioid abuse generally) is so common, how it could happen to anyone, how it could happen to you. Simultaneously, these very same celebrity and public qualities allow the narrative to remain on the level of the exceptional: an opioid overdose is an exceptional moment; it is an uncommon moment (drawing on the uncommonness of celebrity); as exceptional and uncommon, such an instance may become momentarily hypervisible but will ultimately remain in the realm of the unknown and invisible.

Furthermore, inasmuch as figures like Prince, Phillip Seymour Hoffman, Heath Ledger, Cory Monteith, and others have become emblematic of contemporary American pop culture, contextualizing opioids in the bodies of these figures serves to situate the event of an overdose specifically, and opioids gener-

50 Jennifer Ludden, "An Even Deadlier Opioid, Carfentanil, is Hitting the Streets," *National Public Radio,* September 2, 2016, http://www.npr.org/sections/health-shots/2016/09/02/492108992/an-even-deadlier-opioid-carfentanil-is-hitting-the-streets.

51 David Armstrong, "Dope Sick," *STAT,* August 2, 2016, https://www.statnews.com/feature/opioid-crisis/dope-sick/.

52 Tom Howell, Jr., "Opioid Epidemic Demands Greater Access to Key Medications: Govt. Report," *The Washington Times,* October 27, 2016, http://www.washingtontimes.com/news/2016/oct/27/opioid-epidemic-demands-access-key-meds-report.

ally, as emblematic of American culture and as an undercurrent of this specific moment. The opioid epidemic is people we know dying. The opioid epidemic is people we value for their contributions to our culture dying.

By maintaining the language of exceptionality that celebrity allows for, narratives utilizing this rhetorical move express a conceptualization of opioids as a "social injury…[that is] individually culpable rather than that which symptomatizes deep political distress."[53] These narratives are able to state, on the one hand, the feeling of people doing this to themselves, something we each have to avoid on our own and, on the other hand, an idea of "our culture" doing this to itself as a historic expression of dissolution. The opioid epidemic and a moment of overdose become situated within these narratives as a uniquely American political situation and feeling. Buried under these feelings, the guise of celebrity and focus on the individual (death) is the "deep political distress" such moments are representative of.

It would also be important at this point to acknowledge an additional and related set of statistics to those that make up the opioid epidemic. In the first half of 2016, a number of articles appeared with headlines that were generally variations on the question, "Why Are So Many White Americans Dying?" These articles came in response to a set of data released showing a general rise in the death rates for middle class, middle-aged, and lower-educated white Americans; a rise of 11% since 2000. This stands in contrast to a decrease in death rates seen for both African American (-23%) and Hispanic (-14%) populations. The rise was fueled mainly by deaths attributed to poisonings (overdoses), chronic liver disease (i.e., as seen in alcoholism), a rise in suicide rates, and obesity (and related diseases).[54] One of the most striking explanations given for this is that of reference group theory. Essentially, this theory states that it is not only objective parameters of recent history, like those outlined above,

53 Wendy Brown, *States of Injury: Power and Freedom in Late Modernity* (Princeton, NJ: Princeton University Press, 1995), 27.
54 Andrew J. Cherlin, "Why Are White Death Rates Rising?" *The New York Times,* February 22, 2016, http://www.nytimes.com/2016/02/22/opinion/why-are-white-death-rates-rising.html.

that influence current situations and individual behaviors but feelings about this history (and, specifically, how it compares to now) that are generating patterns of behavior. Or, to rephrase: whether you think of your current moment, and the moment your community, state, or country is in, is better or worse than the moment and experience of your parents' generation will influence your individual behavior in such a way as to generate political, social, and economic structures.[55] The opioid epidemic is that nothing is what it used to be.

Reference group theory, or reference group theory offered as an explanation for a rise in white death rates, reinforces the reading that the rhetorical move of "opioids contextualized in the bodies of famous people" is a representation of feelings of a loss of culture (and concurrent, previous, political, social, and economic structures) while also providing a secondary interpretation. By focusing on figures who are not only emblematic of American culture but who have become emblematic of specific time periods (i.e., Prince and the 1980s), this rhetorical move gestures to a sense that *this is what history feels like*; that this ongoing crisis-time of loss is one of and within history, and what is and will be historic about now. The opioid epidemic is what it will be.

23 Years Old

On average, the majority of current opioid users are 23 years old. As with any age, being both a length of time and quality of time (i.e., young is a temporal quality distinct from old as a temporal quality) set within a larger timeframe (history), "23" names a way that history becomes contextualized within and as a *lifetime*. "23" names the quality and experience of being 23 years old within this specific historic and historical moment, while living in, with, and under all of the specific parameters discussed above.

What distinguishes 23 from other ages is a distinct sense of liminality. The liminality of being 23 is so striking, and so different from other ages, that this time of life has recently been categorized as a new developmental stage: emerging adulthood.

55 Cherlin, "Why Are White Death Rates Rising?"

Emerging adulthood is defined as the period from 18 years old up to one's 30s, though generally ending in the mid-20s, and is characterized by identity explorations, instability, feeling in-between, maintaining a focus on oneself, and a sense of wide-open possibilities.[56] Emerging adulthood is, above all, a time of these possibilities. While the relationship of this developmental stage to historically less privileged populations is contested within the literature, inasmuch as actualizing certain possibilities or having the time to explore widely is limited by socioeconomic and disability-related factors, the very fact that "emerging adulthood" exists is illustrative of how 23 does not fit into other preexisting social or developmental categories. By being in-between on these multiple levels, 23 is a boundary moment, regardless of socioeconomic position: whether you have been working since high school or are just graduating from a four-year degree program, 23 is a moment of establishing independence and of having to come out into a world, while at the same time (if possible) "trying everything," "doing whatever you want," and fully taking advantage of that "world of possibilities." However, for those who are 23 years old now, these popular discourses surrounding age are set in a political and economic context of ongoing and deep recession that has seen not only high levels of unemployment, especially among younger people, but also a distinct shift towards a freelance, sharing, and gig-based economy in which historic job categories are dissolving; how do you establish financial independence in an economic moment with few jobs and fewer livable wages? Additionally, many of the jobs that are available (including both specialized fields like technology or within the creative economy, as well as part-time or temporary low-level staff positions) require a higher degree, which for many entails an also higher degree of debt — a debt that would be just coming into effect at 23. Seeking alternatives, people may turn to sectors of the economy that have historically required only a high school degree or trade certificate, like manufacturing work. But throughout the recession, and coupled to both an economic

56 Jeffrey Jensen Arnett, *Emerging Adulthood: The Winding Road from the Late Teens through the Twenties* (Oxford: Oxford University Press, 2004), 9.

shift towards gig-based work as well as larger trends in outsourcing, globalization, and automatization, the number of such jobs available has markedly declined. By being a boundary moment of coming out into a world *within* this specific economic context, and especially inasmuch as it contrasts both popular narratives or expectations of being able to do everything as well as historic employment statistics, "23 years old" names the moment at which it may become apparent that it is no longer as good for you as it was for your parents.

In proximity to the opioid epidemic and addiction generally, "23" names an additional moment of contrast. The liminality of being 23 years old and its standing as a boundary moment extends to the narratives age-related expectations get rhetorically funneled into. "23" names a group of people about whom existing narratives of healthcare, addiction, and dependency are no longer fully relevant or fitting. The experience, social position, and trajectory of a person in the zone of addiction at 23 cannot be understood under a "save our children" narrative any more than it can be understood within "adults taking responsibility for themselves." "23" can be read as naming both of these narratives while at the same time naming its own disjuncture from them. And this is not solely a rhetorical matter, but effects legal and health policy. For instance, under the Affordable Care Act, a person can remain on their parents' health insurance policy (which may or may not, most likely may not, cover addiction treatment) until age 26; at the same time, there is an entrenched set of social expectations about how, by 26, one is supposed to have achieved, at the least, financial independence and full employment if not also be in some stage of beginning one's own family. Even as these norms are changing, the existing narratives lack adequate descriptions.

This is the liminality of the mass. This is a mass that stands in contrast to that of the AIDS epidemic. In the 1970s, there was no question (within mass media and popular discourse) about the marginal and outsider status of gay men. Now, "23" names a core confusion about how to understand *who* the opioid epidemic is: where does the mass fit? Is "mass" even an applicable word, or should these people be situated along a (safe, distanced) proximity? How do we understand and name populations that fail to fit into preexisting ideas about social structure and individual behavior, beyond the terms that have been used frequently ("millennial," or descriptors of grown children who "boomerang" to their family home again) but remain inadequate, for they fail to acknowledge the larger picture: the very idea of a *liminality of the mass* demands attention to an overarching confusion over normative categorizations, beyond any that are age- or socioeconomic-specific. Because if this many people, this mass, is so liminal while remaining, literally, *the average,* where is the epidemic and what does it actually consist of? If whiteness is ultimately about feelings of cultural loss and loss of privilege, "23" names a feeling of confusion, and confusion at the loss of normative categories.

Rural

Outside of the ongoing narratives surrounding the rural nature of the opioid epidemic, outside, even, the specifics of the statistics themselves (apart from a general prevalence), how can we begin to better understand and re-contextualize what rural is? That is, taking as a basic fact the concentration of opioids within rural environments more so than urban ones, as a measure of the sheer quantity of the combination of deaths, people, and substances, what other things can we learn about what rural is outside of the *why is this happening, here* trend within opioid epidemic coverage; such a trend converges with aforementioned discussions of whiteness.

I ask these questions especially as someone who does not live in a rural or suburban area, but in Boston. This is actually my only point of departure from the other demographic averages of the opioid epidemic. What does the rural mean when set always at a distance? On the one hand, there are socioeconomic assumptions built into this very question, that get further perpetuated with every expression of exactly this feeling of distance: that there is some actual distance, like a distance produced by a population that is so far from normative, between myself, or the Northeast, and that of populations living in rural America. I am most interested in how this very sense of distance becomes the way in which "rural" takes on meaning within popular narratives.

And within other fields: there is a long history within philosophy and modernist theory of notions of the urban, and the social, psychological, and political nature of an urban environment. How can we understand the rural within the terms set up by such work, or in contrast to them? Classically, within the work of theorists such as Walter Benjamin and Jean Baudrillard, the urban is figured as a site of disconnection, anonymity, and extreme disorientation brought on particularly by a simultaneous heightening and dissolving of the senses, itself a product of being within an environment where simulacra and simulations (and concurrent technological developments) are so heavily concentrated. The urban ultimately becomes a cipher for the failures of the modern nation state and society and the dangers of immersion in a technological futurity; these systems are most often at work in producing such feelings of disorientation and disconnection. The urban comes to function as an almost dystopia. In contrast, the rural, while rarely theorized, remains within popular discourse as an idyllic, peaceful environment where *everything has remained as it should.* Such sentimental renderings of the rural can be seen especially in the recent and ongoing trends within media and consumerism focused on all things "natural," whether a healthy lifestyle, a move out of the city, self-reliance, and an overall huge spike in interest in lifestyle practices that are actually or are thought to be representative of "how it used to be done." The rural is a site of fantasy, a fantasy into which urban disenchantments (whether within modernist theory or not) are funneled.

But is this actually what the rural becomes if remaining in relation to notions of the urban within theory? Or, can it be read more simply as an opposite: if the urban is a site of anonymity, the rural becomes an atmosphere of a deeply personal reality (also as opposed to simulacra), where everyone knows everyone else, where everyone knows someone who has died within the opioid epidemic. In short, an atmosphere characterized by "high social cohesion and lack of anonymity."[57] This is not better or worse, or

57 Jennifer Sherman, "Rural Poverty: The Great Recession, Rising Unemployment, and the Under-utilized Safety Net," in *Rural America in a Globalizing World: Problems and Prospects for the 2010s,* eds.

more or less accurate, than existing notions of the urban, simply different. Nor is the rural a space exempt from occurrences of or a sense of violence that is often an embedded subtext in popular discourses of the urban, most frequently expressed as fears about gang violence, "bad neighborhoods," or anonymous attacks. Yet article after article within opioid epidemic coverage that focuses on the subset of data pertaining to the general rise in death rates for whites, focusing on small rural towns, documents incidence after incidence of small violence: towns which are seeing a succession of deaths, people all involved in some form of substance abuse and to whom any combination of theft, accident, or family tragedy has happened. It is almost as if the simple fact of (seemingly) everyone knowing someone who has died minimizes each incident; the opioid epidemic is what it is. And it is what it will be: in contrast to the de- or multi-temporalized nature of the urban, the rural becomes a place of an always present, yet within the opioid epidemic, the rural becomes the present of an impossible future; a present caught in the repetition of an addiction, underemployment, or violence, or a present that becomes an expression of an understanding that "rural populations will likely continue to experience hardships into the next decade."[58] This last observation is supported by several years of socioeconomic data that demonstrates that not only have unemployment and poverty rates been higher in rural areas than urban ones for decades, but by 2010, "nonmetropolitan unemployment rates…[had] reached high levels not seen in more than twenty-five years."[59] The recession of the 2000s came deeply into rural areas, and as such communities are generally already lacking in employment opportunities, a qualified workforce, educational resources, and private and governmental support systems, signs of recovery have come much more slowly than they have for larger metropolitan areas. More than in age, which is temporary, and more than in whiteness, which is tied to a somewhat different set of historical structures, precarity and poverty are concentrated in the rural.

Conner Bailey, Leif Jensen, and Elizabeth Ransom (Morgantown: West Virginia University Press, 2014), 532.

58 Sherman, "Rural Poverty," 528.

59 Sherman, "Rural Poverty," 523.

What is striking is how many different ways there are to measure and describe precarity in these areas: not only unemployment and poverty statistics, but in subtle differences within the forms of unemployment that are distinctive of rural areas, and seen in interaction with aforementioned factors like globalization and sector shifts within the economy. For instance, despite some gains that have been made in increasing rural employment in the years post-recession, the overall poverty rates and wages remain down. An explanation for this lies in the fact of which jobs (mainly manufacturing) were lost within the recession and due to globalization and outsourcing and the growth, in turn, of the service sector, made up of care, hospitality, and similar jobs. Men, generally, lost manufacturing jobs; women, generally, take jobs in the service sector. Lower wages for service sector jobs, especially given lower rates of unionization among service workers, is compounded by the fact that women consistently do not earn as much as men.[60] Furthermore, for any number of reasons, from long commutes without adequate public transportation to social stigma and unfillable work requirements that prevent families from receiving government assistance (as frequently as do families in urban areas),[61] rural areas can be characterized by a lack of help. This lack spreads precarity. In these areas, in particular, precarity easily spreads "beyond effects of specific global events and macroscale structures [and] inhabits the microspaces of everyday life."[62] Furthermore, such a view corresponds accurately to formative 20th-century sociological accounts of addiction, like those researched and written by Chicago-school sociologist Bingham Dai. Through his fieldwork, Dai found that "addiction was likely to be most prevalent in an environment 'in which individuals live mostly by and for themselves, in which the amount of social control is reduced to the minimum, and

60 See Sherman, "Rural Poverty," and Cynthia B. Struthers, "The Past is the Present: Gender and the Status of Rural Women," in Bailey et al., *Rural America in a Globalizing World,* 489–505.

61 Sherman, "Rural Poverty," 531.

62 Nancy Ettlinger, "Precarity Unbound," *Alternatives: Global, Local, Political* 32, no. 3 (2007): 319–40, at 319, https://doi.org/10.1177/030437540703200303.

in which opportunities for unrestrained dissipation and various forms of personal disorganization abound.'"[63] Like the rural in contemporary America, in which individuals live mostly by and for themselves (finding it difficult to activate social support networks within an overall lack of infrastructure, shifting family and gender roles, and stigma attached to a lack of anonymity); in which social control is reduced to a minimum (illustrated, in one sense, by the overall lower rates of welfare receipt in rural as opposed to urban areas); and the opportunities for dissipation abound (because this is the opioid epidemic and this is what it will be — because everything is dissipating).

This precarity, a feeling of its proximity, becomes condensed in another generic rhetorical device of opioid epidemic coverage: the device of *another local. Another local* names all of the news reports that begin with or include any variation on the following phrases: *another local high school student; another local community member; another local teenager; another local family.* What follows such phrases is a summary of another recent and local arrest, overdose death, or incident of drug-related crime. *Another local* becomes another way of saying "epidemic," so as to also concurrently name a sense of precarity unique to the personal, always present nature of the rural: it names a quantity (another, a mass, a growing mass) in a single place (local, here) and the quality of that quantity. Ours.

But if one were to look more specifically at contributing macroscale structures in relation to rural America, what information about the opioid epidemic would there be? How has it happened, broadly, that opioids are so heavily concentrated within these areas? How has this become ours? By looking more closely at the landscape itself, and seeing there a wide open space along river valleys (such as the Ohio River Valley, an early and continuing epicenter), we can see a pattern useful for understanding the globalized network of opioids deeply entangled in rural communities and America generally. Or, rural America is an illustration of and effect of contemporary opioid drug traf-

---

63 Bingham Dai, quoted in Caroline Jean Acker, *Creating the American Junkie: Addiction Research in the Classic Era of Narcotic Control* (Baltimore, MD: Johns Hopkins University Press, 2002), 193.

ficking, the domestic and international policies related to this drug trafficking, and their history.

Historically, opium has been an important cash crop and trade good for centuries, with Afghanistan and parts of Southeast Asia being the world's largest opium producers. This production emerged both because of historic imperial patterns of economic subjugation that saw high demand for opium (and was concurrent with and related to the colonial trade patterns and demand for other substances, from cotton to sugar), and the perpetuation of such economically driven foreign policies into the 20th and 21st centuries, as well as because opium poppies are simply a crop particularly well suited to being grown in arid areas (say, war-torn countries; say, Afghanistan from the 1980s until the 2000s) that are cheap to grow and easy to transport.[64] Heroin production, a next step along an opioid production line, then takes place generally in adjacent areas before being distributed within consuming countries. For the United States, the production-to-distribution pipeline was, throughout the 20th century, a simplified pipeline of Turkey-Marseilles-New York, with additional heroin coming in from Mexican and Colombian traffickers as well. However, Nixon's War on Drugs, initiated in the 1970s, disrupted this pipeline and did succeed in reducing incoming heroin through these channels, but also further opened a global market to organized criminal activities in illicit substances. Similar to the policies detailed in the 1999 *National Drug Control Strategy,* the repressive tactics focusing on production during the 1970s did not produce long-lasting, positive effects, largely because of the unrecognized elasticity of the drug market: "With such elastic constraints, the baton of repression becomes instead a prod

---

64 See David T. Courtright, *Forces of Habit: Drugs and the Making of the Modern World* (Cambridge, MA: Harvard University Press, 2002); Paul R. Blakemore and James D. White, "Morphine, the Proteus of Organic Molecules," *Chemical Communications* 11 (2002): 1159–68, https://doi.org/10.1039/B111551K; and Richard Davenport-Hines, *The Pursuit of Oblivion: A Global History of Narcotics* (New York: W.W. Norton, 2004).

pushing consumption and production in ever-widening spheres and compounding the global drug problem."[65]

It is entirely conceivable that this dissolution of historic opioid trafficking patterns has contributed to the diversity of trafficking being seen within the opioid epidemic now; in addition to afore-mentioned domestic policies built on racial discrimination that have been implemented within the War on Drugs, this change in trafficking as a result of international policies names another way that the War on Drugs could have contributed to the current situation. Currently, with the diversity in trafficking in mind, it is possible to conceive of the opioid epidemic as ultimately *an epidemic of three distinct drugs*: prescription pills, heroin, and other (stronger) synthetic opioids related to fentanyl. As for the patterns in trafficking itself, the DEA identifies "pharmacy theft, fraudulent prescriptions, and illicit distributions by patients and registrants [i.e., medical professionals]" as a main contrib-uting factor in the distribution of prescription painkillers.[66] Continuing trafficking from Mexican and Colombian cartels accounts for much of the heroin being found in the US drug market currently: the United States is in fact the world's largest consumer of Mexican and Colombian heroin.[67] Other synthetic opioids are both manufactured by illicit labs within the United States and Mexico, but are also being produced overseas. To cite the DEA once more, "Overseas labs in China are mass-producing fentanyl and fentanyl-related compounds, and marketing them to drug trafficking groups in Mexico, Canada, and the United States."[68] Much of this trade is conducted anonymously over the Internet; fentanyl itself, related substances, and pill-manufactur-ing equipment can be bought online, generally from China, and

65 McCoy, "From Free Trade to Prohibition," 312.

66 Drug Enforcement Agency (DEA), "Fentanyl," December 2016, https://www.deadiversion.usdoj.gov/drug_chem_info/fentanyl.pdf.

67 Central Intelligence Agency (CIA), "The World Factbook: Illicit Drugs," n.d., https://www.cia.gov/library/publications/the-world-factbook/fields/2086.html.

68 DEA, "DEA Report: Counterfeit Pills Fueling U.S. Fentanyl and Opioid Crisis," July 22, 2016, https://www.dea.gov/divisions/hq/2016/hq072216.shtml.

shipped relatively anonymously.[69] The anonymity of such a process is striking when thought in conjunction with the products these processes are primarily producing: counterfeit pills. That is, much of the fentanyl being brought into the United States is processed into forms that look identical to popularly abused prescription drugs, like OxyContin, which sell at higher prices than fentanyl or heroin. The recent, and huge, rise in overdose deaths can be directly linked to this cycle of anonymity and counterfeit facades: people who take these fake pills, not knowing or understanding the presence of fentanyl and other highly potent substances within them, can easily die of an accidental overdose. Because, to be clear, fentanyl and specifically related forms such as carfentanil, which is thousands of times more potent than morphine, can be so dangerous that it is possible to inhale or absorb through the skin a lethal amount. In fact, carfentanil is so deadly that it has been the subject of chemical warfare research in multiple countries, including the United States, and is now banned under the Chemical Weapons Convention. "Counterfeit pills" becomes a cipher for the unknown–invisible qualities of the opioid epidemic. So invisible, so unknown, so quiet and anonymous, that these qualities can extend even to the substances themselves.

Carfentanil has recently been responsible for contributing not only to this general and ongoing rise in overdose rates, but also to a series of specific events, days and weekends, in which single towns are seeing numbers of overdoses previously unseen and unheard of. In these deaths, its mass, and the global networks of distribution it is related to and embedded in, carfentanil is emblematic of an ongoing and historical pattern of multiple progressions within opioid use. On the simplest level, it represents a progression frequently reported among opioid users, who start by abusing prescription pills before moving onto heroin, and then onto even stronger synthetic substances from there. This progression mirrors a much longer history of the transition that opioids have made from natural to synthetic, and simultaneously from less to more potent. This history began with opium

69 Ludden, "An Even Deadlier Opioid, Carfentanil, Is Hitting the Streets."

poppy production, wherein a sap harvested from the poppies was eaten (producing a much slower and less potent high than anything seen now) and moved from there to the practice of smoking opium, to the development of laudanum and other medical tinctures of morphine and herbal ingredients, to the isolation of the molecule of morphine (by Emmanuel Merck, of the pharmaceutical company of the same name) and the development of intravenous and hypodermic technologies for injecting morphine from the 1830s to the 1850s, to the development of heroin, a synthetic opioid, by the pharmaceutical company Bayer in 1897. The 20th century then saw the development of the more modern class of synthetic opioids, many of which were produced either within or just after wars (as was methadone, discovered by German scientists during WWII) or through government-funded research (as performed at the US Narcotic Farm in the 1930s, a prison and drug treatment center in which the US government developed and tested drugs on addicts/prisoners, including many still commonly in use today, such as Dilaudid, Demerol, and codeine).[70] Throughout this progression, as each form made morphine more and more accessible, physiologically, opioids became more and more potent. What produces the euphoric effects of an opioid is the morphine (or morphine-derived) molecule within it; the more easily and quickly this morphine is able to attach to opioid receptors in the body and brain, the more quickly and strongly euphoric effects (as well as analgesic effects) will be felt. Thus, the time it takes for digestion slows the high of eating opium, but a strong synthetic opioid injected directly into the bloodstream will make more morphine available, faster. This progression is a progression of potency concurrent with desire: if laudanum was enough, why develop intravenous morphine? If morphine was enough, why search for stronger forms? If heroin was enough, why import stronger, deadlier synthetics? At the same time, this is not a desire in the usual sense of it, or

70 For an overview of opioid production history, see Courtright, *Forces of Habit*; Davenport-Hines, *The Pursuit of Oblivion*; Blakemore and White, "Morphine, the Proteus of Organic Molecules;" Quinones, *Dreamland*; and Markus Heilig, *The Thirteenth Step: Addiction in the Age of Brain Science* (New York: Columbia University Press, 2015).

desire alone. Opioids, like other pharmaceutical and natural substances (from caffeine and sugar to nicotine and cocaine) produce physical tolerances in those who use these substances: in order to attain subsequent highs (or subsequent levels of pain relief, energy, satiety, and so on, in relation to these and other substances) more and more of the opioid must be taken. The drive towards accumulation produced by physical tolerance is and is not desire and could be referred to, almost in shorthand, as addiction itself, as the emotional and biological dialectic that fuels addiction. Yet an entire global history could be written of a communal drive towards *more*, of any substance; why single any individual person, individual population, or individual substance out as being any different from this larger pattern? For moral reasons alone? Because it can be difficult to see how the concept of "personal values," as pertaining to a sense of morality, intersects deeply with the values implicit in historic and current political economic situations?

The relationship with China embedded in this network of newer synthetics similarly mirrors an earlier point in the history of opioids and their role in international economies. Specifically, this relationship calls to mind the Opium Wars fought in the 1800s, which Britain pursued with the aim of keeping China's borders open to trade in opium, a crop hugely profitable for Britain through its production in British colonial India. "Drug taxation was the fiscal cornerstone of the modern nation state."[71] These wars took place amid an era of policy focused on free trade. It was only during the 20th century that the United States and a post-war League of Nations led a turn towards complete prohibition, culminating in the War on Drugs of the 1970s until today, as discussed. If the China of the 1800s that was involved in the Opium Wars is representative of a policy era focused on free trade, the relationship to China and opioid distribution today is emblematic of a drug trafficking network that has emerged in direct response to the policy progression from trade to prohibition: a move to Internet-dependent forms of trafficking, a move towards complete anonymity, demonstrates a progression of opioid trafficking into deeper and blacker markets. It does not mat-

71 Courtright, *Forces of Habit,* 15.

ter how many wars have been or can be fought; whether these wars are perceptible acts of violence or acts of policy, opioids will remain in production, will remain economically and physically desirable, and will remain in circulation. The opioid epidemic is what it will be.

Substance

With an understanding of this matrix of social, political, economic, and personal conditions in place, how can we come to understand the substance at the heart of this matrix and at the center of these globalized networks? What are opioids? What are painkillers? What is a substance? On the simplest level, opioids are substances derived from or related to the opium poppy, *Papaver somniferum,* and specifically to the chemicals found in the sap of that poppy: thebaine (from which codeine is derived) and morphine, most importantly. Opioids are also all synthetic chemicals that are derived from morphine or based on more recently isolated molecules within the same class. Opioids are morphine, codeine, hydrocodone, heroin, hydromorphone, meriperidine, oxycodone, naloxone, fentanyl, carfentanil, tramadol, methadone, buprenorphine, Suboxone, Demerol, Vicodin, Percocet, Lortab, Zohydro, Lorcet, Norco, Dilaudid, OxyContin, Ultram, Opana, Buprens, Actiq, Fentora, Duragesic, Dolcet, Durotep, Fentanest, Fentanil, Fentanilo, Haldid, Jurnista, Leptanal, Nobligan, OneDuro, Sublimaze, Sufenta, Tramaxet, Tramal, Ultracet, Vivitrol, Avinza, Embeda®CII, Tussigon®ER, Troxyca®ER, Movantik, Moventig, Contrave.

By taking into account all of the physical objects opioids are as well as the social, political, economic, and biological forces they are bearers of, I would define *substance* within Marxist terminology as a commodity and product of commodification. Doing so allows for the retention of all of these aspects within a sense of what an opioid is, as "for Marx…a commodity is never just a commodity but, as the result of the complex and dissimulating activity of *commodification,* always remains itself a social force as well as the condensed site of social forces."[72] Opioids,

72 Brown, *States of Injury*, 13.

and a *substance* generally, thus names a material object as well as the above sites of social condensation (i.e., whiteness, being 23 years old, a rural community) and, furthermore, includes the *residues this condensation leaves,* and the residues left by unseen or unidentified further social forces. For Marx, "commodities are residues of the products of labor."[73] Here I would shift away from a sense of substance-as-commodity, in solely Marxist terms, because in a substance as proliferate as opioids, what is labor? What, exactly, is human or socially necessary (the "socially necessary labor" of Marx) within the objects of opioids? Is an opioid a product, or is it also always itself productive? In producing biological effects, whether through addiction or pain treatment, is an opioid one product or many? What becomes residual? The residues, or traces, or imperceptible or perhaps simply subjective effects of an encounter with or proximity to opioids may also include such social forces as: the history of drug control policy, as outlined (leaving as residue the number of incarcerated people it is currently and has been responsible for, the way taxes paid by American citizens, paid by you, are put toward the costs of this war); the colonial policies enacted through and because of opium (leaving as residue physical traces on the landscapes of places like Afghanistan, and the effects these traces had throughout 20th- and 21st-century international policies concerning Afghanistan); the pricing and marketing strategies of pharmaceutical companies (litigation becoming the residue of aggressive marketing in the cases of companies like Purdue Pharma's marketing of OxyContin); the racial discrimination that unevenly distributes these substances throughout neighborhoods (the differences in pain epidemiology, as directly linked to racism systemic within medicine, is a residue of opioids); and on and on, into and including the biological. Aspects of the biological forces condensed into and emerging in response to opioids will be detailed much more clearly in subsequent sections, but for now I'll add to these existing residues: changes in dopamine levels; changes to the frontal cortex through repeated opioid abuse; the neu-

---

73 Karl Marx, quoted in David Harvey, *A Companion to Marx's Capital* (New York: Verso, 2010), 18.

roanatomy of chronic pain; liver toxicity; and central nervous system depression.

As a substance constituted, always, by a deeply entangled biosocial nature such as this, one can only ever be in relationship to both what is social and what is biological about and in such a substance, simultaneously. *Material proximity* is a way to name exactly a biosocial relationship to a biosocial substance. A material proximity can be constituted as a physical, medical, legal, emotional, economic, psychological, and intellectual experience through and as such concepts as use/abuse, treatment, licit/illicit, what is life-saving, what is life-threatening, pain/relief, what is overwhelming, what is surprising, what becomes a habit; in other words, through many of the ways we have for understanding how a substance can be positioned in relation to your body. And while, again, material proximity will be defined in more detail in coming chapters, what is important to note now about such a relationship, and the very term itself, is that this is not only a distance. *Proximity* is a kind of distance beyond simply length. It is always already a relationship between two things. Proximity is a distance you are *in*. Given this, and given also the proliferation of opioids physically, within the environment, and socially and biologically within bodies and across history, it should be clear that opioids are a substance so dense, so rhizomatic, so epidemic, that it is absolutely possible to be in a material proximity to them *even when you think you are at a slight remove.*

If one can be in and maintain a material proximity to opioids without even being consciously or cognitively aware of such a relationship, how can it be said that any material proximity is truly and entirely a matter of choice? If a material proximity can also equally apply to any substance, to the substances you do choose to be with (the chocolate you eat, the coffee you choose to drink every morning, the cotton of the sheets you prefer) and including also, implicitly, proximities you are unaware of because of the way certain aspects of the physical environment are routinely taken for granted (the industrial agriculture and history of colonialism residual in the chocolate, coffee, and cotton you choose) and extending to the physical environment of one's own body, aspects of which are also routinely taken for granted (as in the fact, for instance, that digestive enzymes, blood sugar, stomach acid, the calcium and sodium ions producing nerve signals, and so on are all material substances in especially deep proximity to your body — and, as in the case of manufactured insulin or digestive enzymes from animal sources linked to industrial agriculture practices, even such seemingly pure biological materials also contain social residues), than how is it possible to categorize, accurately, such relationships along a rubric of only choice or not a choice?

Which is really to say: the people enmeshed in, experiencing, contributing to, and being shaped or informed by the residues and substances of "white, 23 years old, rural" are in material proximities and attachments to the substance of opioids in ways that have come to be understood through the matrices of use/abuse, criminal/citizen, licit/illicit, and pain/desire, but neither the proximity itself nor the conceptualization of it within these ideas fully account for why a proximity alone should be understood as and defined by a moral failure. Addiction is one of many possible proximities within the opioid epidemic. My own proximity as a pain patient is also just another possibility. The breadth of possibility for our proximities to and our places within all of the conditions of this epidemic as outlined above should demonstrate that this is not, at any level, an epidemic of individual choices. It is an epidemic that has happened and has come to be understood as such because of and within an affective-political structure of disbelief, loss, liminality and confusion, precarity and unceasing poverty, globalization and failed drug control policies, and pain and desperation. None of these conditions will be adequately or at all met by treating those caught in deep proximity to them as instances of moral and individual failure. The only truly moral issue within the opioid epidemic is the number of people who have died in the time it has taken me to write this.

2

Addiction

Neuroscience

With this understanding of the spatial and social dimensions of a material proximity to opioids in place — conceptualized as addiction and grounded in the social, political, economic, and personal — how can we add an understanding of the temporal dimensions of the same proximity? Or, how does a material proximity to opioids as structured by particular timeframes come to be conceptualized as *addiction*? This is a question about feelings, feelings over time, the feeling of time, and what *takes place* in and across time: addiction within the opioid epidemic is taking place within these discussed political and social dimensions, but these dimensions and the actions and attitudes characterizing them come to take place temporally as well.

Addiction itself is deeply characterized by time, shaped by the patterns of usage of a given individual. Medically and as informed by current neuroscientific understandings, addiction is a relapsing and remitting brain disease. Within popular rhetoric, once an addict, always an addict. In a way perhaps understandable to many pain patients, what is ill in chronic illness is time.

But what, exactly, does this time feel like? And how does a set of actions taking place within specific time periods and generative of further temporal experiences come to be constituted as *addiction,* a definition that takes on legs and moves across medical and legal spheres? On a fundamental level, this is also the question of what it is like to take an opioid. Extending this question more deeply into the biological as well, one can ask what it is like for a body to have taken an opioid. Ethically, it may seem like this question is at a slight remove from the urgencies of the opioid epidemic. Who cares about biology in the face of a raging need for and attention to policy? But just as political impulses and narratives embedded within opioid epidemic coverage traffic in and distort understandings of addiction with legal and medical implications, ongoing biological and specifically neuroscientific understandings of addiction cross into and come to complicate legal and medical policy; the two become compatible and inseparable.

To begin, then, at the most basic level: what happens within a body when an opioid is taken? At this point, it will not matter on a molecular level whether that opioid is taken for pain relief or in seeking a high. When an opioid is taken, it will bind to one of three types of opioid receptors sited throughout the body. Each type produces a slightly different set of effects, and these differences are utilized within both pain medicine and addiction treatment to tailor pain relief or prevent withdrawal. Morphine and its relatives bind to *mu*-opioid receptors, sited throughout the brain stem and spinal cord, and produce the well known effects of pain relief and euphoria as well as instances like respiratory depression, constipation, nausea, and headaches, due to their effect on the central nervous system; instances generally grouped as "side effects."[1] A seemingly innocuous term, these side effects (specifically respiratory depression) are usually what are responsible for causing overdose deaths, as large quantities of opioids can stop breathing and cause cardiac arrest.

---

1   See Markus Heilig, *The Thirteenth Step: Addiction in the Age of Brain Science* (New York: Columbia University Press, 2015), for a general overview of the neurology of opioids.

Whether through main desired effects or side effects, an opioid produces these experiences primarily because of the way it acts on particular neurotransmitters. By inhibiting these neurotransmitters that would themselves otherwise inhibit certain areas of the brain, such as the periaqueductal grey area (PGA) and the ventral tegmental area (VTA), the increased activation of these areas produce feelings of pain relief and euphoria, respectively.[2] The strength of all these main and side effects is determined by a combination of quantity and speed: how much of an opioid is available to be immediately absorbed into the bloodstream will determine the perceived potency of that opioid, and what it feels like to take it. It will feel good, it will feel like relief, it will (later) feel like nausea, it will (possibly) feel like an emergency. It will be emotional.

Even in acting on only these specific systems or brain areas, such activity has farther-reaching bodily effects that become especially apparent over time. An opioid taken repeatedly will produce a distinct set of effects from one taken in a single instance. Just as all opioids will bind to opioid receptors regardless of the intention in ingesting such a substance, all opioids taken repeatedly can create a state of physical dependence. This happens in pain patients as much as in addicts, though it may be much more widely recognized as a facet of addiction than a facet of pain management. It's worth recognizing that this also happens in the use of many other substances as well, as demonstrated in common instances like caffeine-withdrawal headaches. The state of physical dependence itself is neutral; only when it becomes attached to the medical, moral, and legal discourses surrounding addiction does "physical dependence" take on its pejorative dimensions.

At the same time, it is also possible to recognize what are, in fact, unique biological features incurred through the repeated ingestion of stronger, more potent, and faster-acting opioids taken in pursuit of a high. Over time, the repeated activation of

2 Alistair D. Corbett, Graeme Henderson, Alexander T. McKnight, and Stewart J. Paterson, "75 Years of Opioid Research: The Exciting but Vain Quest for the Holy Grail," *British Journal of Pharmacology* 147, no. S1 (2006): S153–S162, https://doi.org/10.1038/sj.bjp.0706435.

the aforementioned neuroanatomical structures, and particularly because of the way these areas are activated by dopamine neurons (with dopamine being a neurotransmitter producing diverse effects across multiple systems), major neurological changes will come to be seen. Repeated and heightened activity amid dopamine neurons and the "reward circuitry" they are embedded in trigger processes that ultimately create changes both within these dopamine-modulated specific systems ("within-systems adaptations") and within secondary neurological systems in response to this heightened activity ("between-systems adaptations"). Activity within dopamine-modulated reward circuitry is immediately felt and intensely rewarding, producing euphoria. In an effort to maintain an affective homeostasis, secondary systems within the brain will initiate processes to bring that brain back to a baseline, normal state. However, as in many homeostatic processes, this "baseline" actually represents something of an overshoot, and serves to create a below-baseline state.[3] Or, the anxiety and depression often seen in withdrawal states or in times following a high trigger the pursuit of further highs, which in turn only ever trigger deeper anxiety and depression, and so on. Addiction is a deeply cyclical disease, down to the level of its pathophysiology. Neuroscientifically, these processes and dopamine-related effects as detailed herein state as much. Within popular rhetoric, addiction is a disease of people becoming caught in a deepening spiral of distress. These are not, ultimately, statements that differ from each other in any substantive way and as such, this example provides a basis for understanding that it is not only the neuroanatomical and chemical changes investigated within neuroscience that form a medical definition of addiction, but that the *perceived outward appearance of neuoroanatomical and chemical changes* overlay fundamental ideas about physical dependence and addictive behavior and, when taken together, are crucial to medical, popular, and legal understandings of addiction. Addiction is a relapsing and remitting brain disease; addiction is what a brain disease that is, morally, what self-inflicted looks like; addiction is scientifically confirmed; addiction is exactly what you thought it was.

3   Heilig, *The Thirteenth Step*, 82.

It becomes crucial, in the aim and context of going beyond the attitudes embedded in circulating narratives and opioid epidemic coverage, to point out the fact that it is only these layers of outward appearance and behavior that distinguish the physical dependence of an addict from the physical dependence of a pain patient. Fundamentally, "the claims of pain medicine about the legitimacy of opiate therapy are not based on an identification of the differences between the neurochemistry of analgesia and the neurochemistry of reward."[4] While neuroscientific explanations of addiction may explain *what* is happening within the brain and body of a person repeatedly ingesting opioids, such models do not explain *why*. And perhaps because they do not explain why, neuroscientific models fail to fully divorce themselves from existing social and morally-inscribed ideas. On the one hand, I can offer an explanation of trigger-induced relapse grounded in neuroscience and the role of brain structures like the amygdala and the ventral visual system. On the other hand, I can say that once an addict, always an addict. Within the vast proliferation of materials and proximities within the opioid epidemic, there is room for both of these statements to be true; they ultimately do not disqualify each other, nor is one truly more correct than the other. There is also room for a critique of neuroscience models while retaining a belief that, in fact, addiction *is* a relapsing and remitting brain disease. Addiction, as a disease so deeply characterized by repetition and cycles, is a disease of multiples.

What such relationships between scientific and popular conceptions of addiction demonstrate is twofold. First, that as social and moral attitudes towards addiction are embedded within scientific understandings and as scientific understandings fuel current policy choices, we have, in the end, not moved away from a politics of morality whatsoever; it has simply become one veiled by the language of "neuroanatomical," and "relapsing and remitting," instead of the "vagrant" and "alkie" of early 20th-century public health officials. The misuse of substances has

4   Helen Keane and Kelly Hamill, "Variations in Addiction: The Molecular and the Molar in Neuroscience and Pain Medicine," *BioSocieties* 5, no. 1 (March 2010): 52–69, at 63, https://doi.org/10.1057/biosoc.2009.4.

always been social inasmuch as it has always been about a social body, and will remain politicized as such until a point at which we can understand biology, understand the pathophysiology of addiction, on what are truly neutral grounds; or as neutral as possible, given that biology is always a thing people do as much as a thing that constitutes those people. That is, until a point at which it is possible to say "once an addict, always an addict," and always already also mean that addiction is a relapsing and remitting brain disease. In using the term *addiction* throughout, I mean to include both of these senses — for better or for worse. After all, "once an addict, always an addict" is no more neutral than the term "junkie." And yet one cannot write the word addiction without also recognizing and including its social, even negative, connotations. In short, I understand addiction as "the individual experience of intolerable levels of suffering [set] among the socially vulnerable (which often manifests itself in the form of interpersonal violence and self-destruction) in the context of structural forces (political, economic, institutional, cultural) and embodied manifestations of distress (morbidity, physical pain, and emotional craving)."[5] Though, it is important to remember, it is not only those historically considered to be "the socially vulnerable" who are entangled within this matrix of abuse in the opioid epidemic.

Secondly, the relationship between neuroscience and popular rhetoric and the compatibility of the two suggests that this is, in a sense, *a deeply intelligible epidemic.* So much lay knowledge already exists surrounding addiction and has seemed, in a way, to have been verified and confirmed by the neuroscience research of the past decade. Whether this knowledge is true or not, whether it is ethical to consider such sentiments true or not, it is circulating nonetheless. The opioid epidemic is something we know.

Is it possible to really know what it feels like without being an addict oneself? I can say "pain relief" and "euphoria," but unless you have taken an opioid in pursuit of the latter or been given one in hopes of the former, unless you have encountered an opioid in a time of medical emergency and pain, or personal

5   Phillipe Bourgois and Jeffrey Schonberg, *Righteous Dopefiend* (Berkeley: University of California Press, 2009), 53.

stress and pain, unless you have witnessed the high of another or the pain and relief of another, is it possible to understand these conditions? How can so much lay knowledge exist surrounding addiction (how, really, can addiction be so common) and yet, in the seeming lack of firsthand experience, what fills that void is only the moral imperative to be responsible for oneself, to Just Say No? How do you know what you are saying no to?

As in the forms of repetition, action, and usage that shape any habit, the times of a deep material proximity to opioids in the form of addiction come to influence larger and longer forms of time and the formation of a lifetime; these times and timing are what it feels like. The time and timing of opioids within the opioid epidemic can be expressed, experienced, and understood through these patterns of use: the time spent finding money; the time spent looking for and buying or selling drugs; the way that a high itself becomes a form of time; the repetitive, gentle, and affirmative or confirming temporal quality connoted by the term "nodding," used by heroin addicts to describe the moments immediately following an injection; the time spent coming down from a high; the time spent in treatment; the time spent waiting for a bed in a treatment center to become available; the time spent in and formed by longer cycles of use, withdrawal, recovery, remission, and relapse; the way that withdrawal can last days, yet cravings for opioids can persist for decades;[6] the way that a drug's effects can last only minutes, hours, or days, yet persist and be continued generationally, as seen in the rising rates of neonatal abstinence syndrome among babies born to mothers who used opioids, a rise of 500% during the 2000s;[7] the way that a high can be instantaneous but side effects last for days; the immediacy with which naloxone can reverse an overdose but the differences in timing between the effects of naloxone and the effects of stronger opioids like fentanyl, which means that a person can slip back

6   Heilig, *The Thirteenth Step,* 170.
7   Nora D. Volkow, "What Science Tells Us About Opioid Abuse and Addiction," National Institute on Drug Abuse (NIDA), January 27, 2016, https://www.drugabuse.gov/about-nida/legislative-activities/testimony-to-congress/2016/what-science-tells-us-about-opioid-abuse-addiction.

into an overdose state even after having been already revived; the thirty minutes it takes for my pain medication to start working; the three hours of pain relief a single pill can give me; the necessity of precisely timing this window within a day; the nausea that begins at two and a half hours; the headache the next day; the year a prescription can last me; the number of minutes, at an hourly rate, I work that become equivalent to the $2.33 I paid for my most recent prescription; the way that, months after first writing this, a single pill no longer provides relief and the same prescription now lasts a month; the way that loss of life due to drug use can be measured as an amount of time (both simply, as in the way that every cigarette smoked has been calculated to represent a loss of 5½ minutes of life, and in more complex ways, as in the way that heroin addicts have a 20 to 50 times greater risk of dying than the general population);[8] the way that the length of an addiction can be measured both in lived years and, in a sense, as a prognosis, with the average active heroin user dying of an overdose within 10 years;[9] the time it has taken for opioid prescribing rates, abuse rates, and overdose rates to, in some cases, double and, in others, more than double; the time it takes for an opioid user to transition from prescription drugs to heroin or other street drugs; the way that the time and timing of an addiction becomes embedded, socially and neurologically, so as to produce and augment a *lifetime*; how lifetime changes can then be measured as the 30, 60, or 90 days spent in a standard treatment program or the sixty months spent in an average drug-related prison sentence; how addiction is a chronic illness.

Social Science

Is this, though, exactly how addiction is understood within the context of medicine? While it may be commonly accepted as a

---

8   Helen Keane, "Smoking, Addiction, and the Making of Time," in *High Anxieties: Cultural Studies in Addiction,* eds. Janet Farrell Brodie and Marc Redfield (Berkeley: University of California Press, 2002), 119.

9   Eli Saslow, "How's Amanda? A Story of Truth, Lies, and an American Addiction," *The Washington Post,* July 23, 2016, http://www.washingtonpost.com/sf/national/2016/07/23/numb/.

disease, most medical definitions pertaining to addiction do not actually use this term, but instead define and rely on concepts of substance abuse or substance dependence. For instance, "the American Psychiatric Association's diagnostic manual does not have an entry under the word *addiction,* and its criteria for identifying substance abuse refer primarily to maladaptive social behaviors caused by 'recurrent substance use,' including, among others, the *political-institutional* category of 'recurrent legal problems.'"[10] While neuroscience may confirm these concepts, medical conceptions of addiction as commonly applied and practiced focus primarily on a set of behaviors, forming addiction as a set of behaviors-as-symptoms and a disease-as-behaviors. Doing so "takes for granted a certain level and style of social functioning, assuming that in the absence of drug use the subject would not be facing problems such as unemployment and poverty."[11] Especially in rural settings that may be underfunded, governmentally neglected, and socially isolated, how is it at all possible to separate this unemployment, poverty, and the small violence of the everyday from addiction? Is unemployment or poverty even a behavior? And when it is considered a behavior that contributes to a disease, is this any different from long-standing ideas about the distribution of diseases among the poor? Which is to say: poor people get sick. Because they're poor. Which is also to imply, as Susan Sontag has written: "Responses to illnesses associated with sinners and the poor invariably recommended the adoption of middle-class values," with such precautions becoming, over time, "part of social mores, not a practice adopted for a brief period of emergency, then discarded."[12] The American Dream of "picking oneself up by the bootstraps," of being/becoming a "heroic survivor," of "making it out of poverty," apply to addiction as much to economics. This Mobius strip of poverty, medical definition, disease, treatment, science, and popular belief directly contributes to aforementioned narrative practices taking place

10 American Psychiatric Association (APA), 1994, quoted in Bourgois and Schonberg, *Righteous Dopefiend,* 28.
11 Keane, "Smoking, Addiction, and the Making of Time," 94.
12 Susan Sontag, *Illness as Metaphor and AIDS and its Metaphors* (New York: Farrar, Straus and Giroux, 1978), 142, 162.

within the opioid epidemic. As seen in the "23 years old" aspect of opioid epidemic coverage, a significant part of explanations for the epidemic are constructed through the idea of reference group theory, of thinking that, now, it is no longer as good for you and your generation as it was for your parents, an idea that is deeply tied to this cycle of behavior and poverty-related moralizing. Using Pierre Bourdieu's concept of symbolic violence, which "refers specifically to the mechanisms that lead those who are subordinated to 'misrecognize' inequality as the natural order of things and to blame themselves for their location in their society's hierarchies,"[13] it becomes clear that it is not just the feeling that now is no longer as good, but the misrecognition of "now" as natural, as one's own fault, as personal, and not actually as the product of decades of systemic inequality, capitalism, and discrimination that allows a generation and group of people to believe that it is their fault. And allows many of those institutionally around that group to believe so as well, and to act on those beliefs.

Beyond the specifics of any singular behavior, both medically and within popular discourse, *addiction* circulates as and around three main beliefs. That is, an addict is someone who (visibly) demonstrates or has experienced: a loss of power; the transformative, "taking over," power of drugs; and is currently situated as both a victim and a perpetrator.

Scientifically, an addict loses power because of the way that aforementioned neuroanatomical and chemical changes become self-perpetuating and create long-term brain states. Under such a model, an addict who continues to engage in self-destructive, risky, or harmful behaviors does so not as an expression of a desire, a social injury, a moment of political or personal distress, or because of anything else that is not a biological fact. This does not, again, explain why that person entered addiction in the first place, but once a loss of power has been experienced, there is no reversal. Perhaps this can only be corrected through a continued, or shifted, loss of power: is it a coincidence that within the treatment model of Alcoholics Anonymous, recovery can only commence after a complete giving up of power to a higher figure?

13   Bourgois and Schonberg, *Righteous Dopefiend,* 55.

This dovetails with the loss of power of the addict as understood socially as well, which happens when or because said person is morally and individually weak and unable to prevent a pattern of behavior from taking place, and taking over. Within this understanding of emphasizing individual weakness, an addict who continues to engage in addictive patterns of use does so because they were always already at odds with mainstream cultural values of individual responsibility. Addiction is a personality trait as much as a disease, or symptomatic of a diseased personality.

Having lost power, the addict then becomes *subject* to the substance at hand, and experiences the transformative power of that substance — its ability to take over. Scientifically and medically, this happens because the substance is able to cause substantive biological changes which then enact and perpetuate further altered states. In short, it is almost more so that these biological changes are the source of a transformative power themselves than any given substance. Because this explanation remains rooted in the physical body of the addict, it is almost as if this simply reiterates the popular belief that if an addict *really* wanted to stop, they would and would be able to; the addict themselves is seen as the problem and the solution. Medical definitions seem to simply transfer the site of this problem from the person to the body (or, specifically, the brain). Such beliefs hold true in the context of other conditions seen as partially or fully constituted by behavior and personality, like obesity, in which an obese person (or any overweight person) should be able to lose the weight if only they *really* wanted to and really had the self-control, regardless of genetic or environmental factors. The body is always something that can and should be overcome. Popularly, the transformative power of a substance is figured not necessarily as biological or neurological changes but as what happens as a person who willfully engages in addictive patterns of use begins to experience powerful cravings and a desire for the substance that they are unable to resist. The body is always something to be overcome, and when it cannot be, disease is always a personal failure.

Having lost power and become subject to the substance itself, the addict comes to be situated as both a victim (of the substance) and as a perpetrator, mainly because it was an individual's fault for having begun the use that began the addiction and because of the criminality of most drug use, distribution, and associated activities. Opioid epidemic coverage focused on small towns and personal stories is full of rhetorical devices underlying and creating this dichotomy, featuring people who "fall into the trap" of an addiction "after a single instance of usage,"[14] or "ordinary kids…who were caught up in…a wave of opioid addiction"[15] — the latter not only signaling the powerless victimhood of those "ordinary kids," but in figuring the opioid epidemic as "a wave," also suggests an overwhelming, inescapable, natural force. Fewer examples may be needed for suggesting the perpetrator aspects of addicts; one need look no further than the term "junkie" to see an addict denigrated and assumed to be a person who, having done this to themselves, now deserves it — whatever "it" may be. Or, in a move that one may attribute more to available space and real estate than to an implicit agenda: the fact that public service announcements concerning the reporting and treating of opioid overdoses have been plastered on trash cans (and only trash cans) around Boston for months.

This victim/perpetrator dichotomy comes to demarcate further aspects of an addict: a "good" addict is one who maintains a particular balance between being a victim and being a perpetrator, especially while behaving in ways that are in line with other desirable narratives like recovery/redemption. To borrow a figure from opioid epidemic coverage, the bodies of famous people illustrate this balance well. In particular, addiction memoirs that become bestsellers are often characterized by exactly this balance of victim/perpetrator. In his memoir *Night of the Gun,* the late journalist David Carr described a single moment that fully encapsulates this dynamic. One night, Carr writes, he left his two young daughters alone, locked in a car on a freezing cold night while he entered a house to buy cocaine. Through the single act of leaving his children in the car, Carr becomes both a perpetrator — though, importantly, the kids ultimately

14 Keane, "Public and Private Practices: Addiction Autobiography and its Contradictions," *Contemporary Drug Problems* 28, no. 4 (2001): 567–595, at 591, https://doi.org/10.1177/009145090102800404.

15 David Armstrong, "Dope Sick," *STAT,* August 2, 2016, https://www.statnews.com/feature/opioid-crisis/dope-sick/.

remained safe — and a victim, as someone who was driven to these lengths by an overwhelming force. On the opposite of this dichotomy would be a figure like Lance Armstrong (or, really, any number of other sports figures at the center of doping scandals) who, despite his previous survival of testicular cancer, found no real standing as a victim throughout the period of scandal surrounding his use of various performance-enhancing drugs; Armstrong became figured solely as a perpetrator. At the same time, perhaps, he has already been forgiven by many of his fans. This is most likely a reflection of the substance in use itself rather than of Armstrong: it is seemingly easier to move on from performance-enhancing drugs (whether steroids or EPO, a substance that acts on the blood oxygen levels of a person) than from hard or street drugs. But this victim/perpetrator dichotomy has farther-reaching effects than determining which memoirs do well and which sports figures have their careers ended. Because situating addiction as a thing that happens to people, *a disease producing victims,* or a thing people do to themselves, *a behavior committed by perpetrators,* determines what policies are seen as responsible, adequate, and fair. Should the opioid epidemic be fought through law enforcement tactics, through harsher drug-related sentences? Is this a war? Or should the focus be on an expansion of medical treatments, distributed widely to those in need? Ultimately, such questions are applicable to how any disease is understood and defined. Is it something that happened, or something you did? Should you be cared for, or care for yourself? Are you a problem or an object of pity? Are these really separate states? What do you deserve?

Is this an epidemic of a disease or an epidemic of a behavior? If the latter, how can we see relationships between the current opioid epidemic and historic instances of the same behavior happening in the same place at the same time? That is, how is it that some instances of group behavior come to be classified as an epidemic, a crisis, and others as an instance of mass hysteria? For an event to later be considered an instance of mass hysteria, there must have been something that remained misunderstood at the time, allowing for instances of behavior to be seen as hysterical — as without true, valid ground, or as caused by some unseen natural or supernatural force. Whether mass hysteria, an epidemic, or a drug war, all instances and their constructs are about the way we understand and come to categorize people's motivations, and situate them within a specific historical context. For instance, within the events of the Salem witch hunts and trials, what remained misunderstood was any event beyond the realm of known science, as well as the rights, standing, or personhood of women, in the context of a "new," unexplored, and unknown land, seemingly full of natural or supernatural powers: such contexts produced a situation in which the behaviors and motivations of some people — mostly women, an already marginal and marginalized group — were classified as being beyond the realm of the normal. This became and perpetuated its own explanation, and the basis for institutional policy, as it were, concentrated mainly on the persecution and killing of those women involved. Within the opioid epidemic, the narratives currently circulating both within mass media and in the governmental and medical responses being taken depict the epidemic as definitely an instance in which people's behaviors and motivations are aberrant or are beyond the realm of the normal, but the multiplicity and conflicting nature of these narratives demonstrates that what that normal is and the specifics of why are not yet agreed upon. How will this be historicized? As another instance of what has happened to a marginal, marginalized, deserving-to-be-marginalized group of people? Just as contemporary accounts of witch hunts frequently forget how common, normal, and understood beliefs about the existence of witches were at the time of such instances, will we forget how actually normal, common, and understood addiction has been?

Figuring those with specific diseases as both victims and perpetrators, and using this dichotomy to blatantly and subtly laud some and denigrate others, is in no way unique to the opioid epidemic, or even to addiction. One does not have to go all the way back to the time of witch hunts to find examples of historic epidemics, especially those that similarly centered on a disease that involved (or seemed to involve) a behavioral component, directly linked to the opioid epidemic via this dichotomy. AIDS is the most recent and prescient example of such an epidemic. Early responses to AIDS were deeply characterized by a victim/perpetrator dichotomy, expressed and enacted through mass media

accounts, government (non-)responses, and medical (mis-)treat-
ment. Nowhere can this rhetoric be seen more clearly than in a
scene near the end of the documentary *How to Survive a Plague.*
Having depicted, through original archival footage, the years of
work, protests, and demonstrations by the AIDS activist collective ACT UP, the documentary shifts to depictions of governmental responses. George H.W. Bush is shown addressing a press
conference following ACT UP actions taken to lobby for more,
faster medical treatments (and research supporting them) to be
made available. Bush responds by talking about the spending the
government has already committed to AIDS research, and then
goes on to ask: regardless of medicine, research, or government, if
there is a behavioral component to getting AIDS, why would you
not simply change the behavior?[16] His statement thus figures the
bodies of the AIDS epidemic both as victims (in need of medical
support and government-funded research) and as perpetrators
(through whose behavior this disease was brought on). The
underlying attitudes of these statements and broader responses
to the AIDS epidemic are that it is the fault of an individual for
having come into contact with a substance, whether a virus or a
drug, but that, once there, the person has become victim to that
substance. This dynamic, I would argue, plays out through the
bodies involved in multiple other ongoing instances of misbe-
havior in relation to substances: from obesity (in which obese
people have come into contact, poorly, with "bad" food and
become, subsequently, a victim to be pitied — though also an
object of common contempt) to black male police violence (the
substance at hand being racial violence itself, assigning or focusing solely on the victimhood of black men providing a rhetorical
way out of having to, instead, responsibly, focus on the racism
and structural violence inherent in the act). Each figures a case of
behavior slightly askew and detached from its structural causes.

What best illustrates this, perhaps, is a statement made by
a recovering heroin addict in the PBS Frontline documentary
Chasing Heroin. Talking about what her life would be like if she
did not have income from dealing drugs, she says that she would

16 David France, dir., *How to Survive a Plague* (New York: Public Square
Films, 2012).

be living "dime bag to dime bag…you know, like pay check to pay check."[17] Having come into contact with a substance — money, heroin — and having become if not exactly a victim of it, at least fully subject to it, one tries to find a mode of living with the least hardship possible (or the least friction through hardship, or the most hustle).

Citizenship

What effects do these ideas have as they move into governmental spheres of law enforcement, legislation, and policy? Or, how does the material proximity of addiction come to be legally inscribed and practiced, much as the mode of living paycheck to paycheck has legal bounds (such as tax bracket implications)? Being based on addiction as a disease-of-behaviors and behaviors-as-symptoms, medical understandings — of addiction as a relapsing and remitting brain disease — are a product of and dependent on understandings of particular forms of time and sets of activities taking place within certain times. Influenced by these understandings, policy enacted within the opioid epidemic is similarly structured by understandings and beliefs about particular forms of time. This can be seen even in relation to opioids generally, as in the practice of writing prescribing guidelines and medication instructions: "Take 1 every 4 to 6 hours," with the legal implication being (or becoming) that taking a medication more frequently is grounds for a determination of abuse. In relation to abuse deterrents specifically, the importance of and reliance on time is seen in multiple instances, such as recently proposed legislation that institutes time limits (of 3 to 7 days) on first-time prescriptions, thereby regulating not only the length of an engagement with opioids, but the length of an engagement at a particular point within a lifetime: the first time. This focus extends throughout recent CDC guidelines, published in March of 2016, that also urge doctors to prescribe for *as short a time as possible,* and only *after* having tried all other available treatments,

17 Frontline, *Chasing Heroin* (Arlington, VA: Public Broadcasting Service, 2016), https://www.pbs.org/wgbh/frontline/film/chasing-heroin/.

all the while instituting *random* drug testing and prescription monitoring of patients.[18]

One of the clearest encounters between medical and legal understandings of addiction as based on time takes place in my own act of taking my medications: it could be something as simple as the number of hours I wait between taking doses of my own medication that would augment my standing as a pain patient to that of a drug abuser, if not addict. Or, augmenting my material proximity to opioids through time would augment my citizenship and the form of citizenship that should remain available to me. As a pain patient, a "good" patient taking medications at appropriate, prescribed doses and times, I am a law-abiding citizen with full access to rights, in direct opposition to the criminal nature of an addict, taking medications too frequently, whose rights should be "appropriately" curtailed — regardless of the fact that the substance in each instance is one and the same, and regardless of the fact that it would not be a matter of possession that changes across these examples, though possession is a criteria for abuse and criminality in the case of nearly all other illicit substances. I can be a law-abiding citizen in possession of illegal substances only when I am using those substances as prescribed and regulated. This is important to acknowledge not only because of what it demonstrates about the ways that citizenship is being shaped by the opioid epidemic but also because this is one of the only instances in which sickness and disability is a privilege. It is being sick itself that allows me to retain my privilege and full citizenship in the context of this epidemic.

These ideas about time, abuse, and citizenship are condensed into ongoing legal responses to the opioid epidemic through the discourses circulating around drug courts and medical maintenance treatment. Both are standard approaches to treating addiction and subsequent or related problems concerning criminal activity. Drug courts create a process in which people who have been arrested on drug-related charges are able to avoid jail time

18 Centers for Disease Control and Prevention (CDC), "CDC Guideline for Prescribing Opioids for Chronic Pain — United States, 2016," *Morbidity and Mortality Weekly Report,* March 18, 2016, https://www.cdc.gov/mmwr/volumes/65/rr/rr6501e1.htm.

by instead agreeing to enter and complete a treatment program, determined by a judge. In general, defendant/addicts who have no history of prior arrests or no history of violent offenses are offered this option. This option is also predominantly available to white people. Because of this standing of drug courts as a treatment-focused, quasi-criminal process, defendant/addicts are figured not as criminals with no rights but as citizens who have retained some rights or some form of freedom — despite being still subject to law, and subject to treatment set by a court. Though drug courts have been in existence since the 1980s, the number of drug courts in the US has doubled in the past decade,[19] rising even within the past several years from 1,504 in 2009 to 2,361 in 2015.[20] These courts serve approximately 120,000 defendant/addicts annually, of whom approximately half fail to graduate.[21] The main arguments in support of drug courts focus on the savings they represent, due to decreased crime and the success rates for graduates. The most frequently cited statistics across governmental sources are those from the National Association of Drug Court Professionals, which note that 75% of graduates remain arrest-free for at least two years following graduation.[22] However, this seemingly high rate is such because it counts only those who successfully completed their mandated treatment program. While it may be true that lowered arrest rates do represent a savings in terms of the cost of processing and housing prisoners, it is also true that "policy analysts have also documented that there was no clear relationship between incarceration rates and decreases in crime, drugs, and violence during the 1990s": that is, during the height of the War on Drugs.[23] The US has the high-

19 Frontline, *Chasing Heroin.*
20 Celinda Franco, "Drug Courts: Background, Effectiveness, and Policy Issues for Congress" (Washington, DC: Congressional Research Service, 2010), https://fas.org/sgp/crs/misc/R41448.pdf.
21 Maia Szalavitz, "How America Overdosed on Drug Courts," *Pacific Standard Magazine,* May 18, 2015, https://psmag.com/how-america-overdosed-on-drug-courts.
22 Massachusetts Judicial Branch, "Drug Courts: Facts and Statistics," 2016, http://www.mass.gov/courts/programs/specialty-courts/drug-courts-facts-and-statistics.html.
23 Bourgois and Schonberg, *Righteous Dopefiend,* 598.

est rate of incarceration in the world, with the average annual cost of housing a single prisoner at almost $24,000; the state of California alone recently spent almost $7 billion in a single year on the cost of processing and housing prisoners, building 53 new prisons within two decades.[24] Especially given that so few avoid jail time despite participation in drug courts, whose quality of life do such practices improve?

Those who fail to complete treatment, and whose failure may have been due to continued substance use or an inability to attend all components of a treatment program, are sent back to court where they are sentenced by a judge, in the absence of a trial or jury, on the basis of the police report of the original incident. This process ensures that the defendant/addict's future citizenship is, from the moment upon entering a drug court, dependent on treatment and therefore on successful subscription to and attainment of medical models of addiction and what "recovery" looks like. When recovery, as figured in the practices of the majority of US drug courts, looks completely substance-free, *material proximity produces citizenship and access to freedom.* "According to a 2012 study, only about a third of all drug courts permit participants to start maintenance as the treatment component of their program, and many oppose it."[25] That is, treatment of opioid addiction with methadone or similar substances is not allowed for the vast majority of participants, despite the fact that methadone maintenance medication has been proven, across multiple measurements, to be the most successful practice for treating an opioid addiction. And these attitudes are not confined to drug courts, but extend into the jails themselves, where maintenance medication is banned at rates even higher than those found in drug courts.[26] This indicates that the treatment programs implemented by drug courts are focused on complete detox and based on therapeutic practices, including talk therapy and support groups. While helpful, these practices alone do not save lives. Nor are such practices based on current, evaluated, and evidence-based medical protocol. They

24 Bourgois and Schonberg, *Righteous Dopefiend,* 596.
25 Szalavitz, "How America Overdosed on Drug Courts."
26 Szalavitz, "How America Overdosed on Drug Courts."

are, ultimately, law enforcement models, not treatment models. In an overview of drug courts, the National Institute of Justice describes the courts as "usually managed by a nonadversarial and multidisciplinary team including judges, prosecutors, defense attorneys, community corrections, social workers, and treatment service professionals."[27] The order of this listing speaks volumes.

Medical maintenance treatment represents an alternative. A subset of governmental responses to the opioid epidemic has involved attention to the distribution of such treatments, which describes a practice of prescribing substances like methadone (but also newer drugs like Suboxone and buprenorphine) to, essentially, remove the presence of heroin or other opioids from a person's life and body. Taking a single dose of such a medication daily prevents the person from going into withdrawal, because these medications bind to opioid receptors as much as heroin does, though they block the effect of any other opioid that may be taken and they do not themselves produce any of the desirable effects, like euphoria, of other opioids: this group of medications is therefore called opioid antagonists. Recently, the government has acted to expand access to these treatments through efforts like raising the limits placed on doctors for how many patients they may treat at one time through maintenance medication. The federal limit is now 200 patients annually per doctor. This may seem like a lot, but it is important to note that not all doctors who qualify to provide such treatment choose to do so. Access to treatment is also compounded by policies like the fact that *any* doctor can prescribe methadone for pain management, but only licensed methadone clinics can dispense it for addiction treatment. Furthermore, what licensed clinics exist are often sited in urban settings, out of reach of the rural foci of the opioid epidemic, and often face strong community opposition throughout any planning or building process, as clinics are usually seen as magnets for criminal activities. This is despite the fact that, according to a 2004 World Health Organization study,

27 National Institute of Justice, "Drug Courts," January 10, 2017, http://www.nij.gov/topics/courts/drug-courts/pages/welcome.aspx.

criminal activity among those who are in their first year of medical maintenance treatment is reduced by about one half.[28]

Medical maintenance treatment represents an alternative that saves lives. Not only is it known to lower the death rate of opioid addiction by 66% to 75%, it also cuts the risk of a fatal overdose (following an initial nonfatal overdose) in half.[29] There are, as with any medication, downsides to consider, like the fact that patients in treatment for opioid addiction pay more for care than patients with abuse related to other drugs,[30] or the onerous nature of having to receive, in person, only a single dose of medication every single day. Given that methadone and other opioid antagonists are extremely potent medications, I am not arguing that they should be distributed in large quantities like other prescriptions; rather, the solution would be more clinics, more doctors, in more locations. Why is this not already the case? Why, really, is it that evidence-based medicine, prized in practically every other field of medical practice, is not the standard for addiction treatment? This has been a systemic elimination of medical maintenance treatment and related practices, generally considered as a model of harm reduction rather than only law enforcement or treatment: "In the mid-2000s, merely using the phrase *harm reduction* disqualified U.S. researchers from receiving federal funding...project officers at the National Institute on Drug Abuse [under George W. Bush] routinely advised researchers to remove the words *condom, needle exchange, sex worker* and *homosexual* from the titles and abstracts of their grant proposals."[31] These practices are an example of the way "the War on Drugs shaped, and continues to shape, the direction of epide-

28 Szalavitz, "How America Overdosed on Drug Courts."
29 Massachusetts Department of Public Health, "Data Brief: An Assessment of Opioid-Related Deaths in Massachusetts, 2013–2014," September 2016, https://www.mass.gov/files/documents/2017/08/31/chapter-55-opioid-overdose-study-data-brief-9-15-2016.pdf.
30 Robin Gelburd, "The opioid epidemic is skyrocketing private insurance costs," *STAT,* September 26, 2016, https://www.statnews.com/2016/09/26/opioid-epidemic-private-insurance-payments/.
31 Bourgois and Schonberg, *Righteous Dopefiend,* 584.

miological public health research."[32] Furthermore, the inclusion within these practices of a focus on terms like "homosexual" and "condom" indicate that the stigma of the AIDS epidemic has attached itself to and influenced not only AIDS research and treatment, but vastly broader research that is now influencing the treatment directions of the opioid epidemic.

The popular discourse surrounding maintenance treatment is similarly full of objections, either because it is seen as "replacing one substance with another" or as failing to "really" treat an addiction. But such objections falter in the face of so many similar substances: insulin, coffee, sugar — or any number of products produced by the weightloss/diet industry devoted to the "you won't believe it's not." Or nicotine patches, which are nothing if not a maintenance treatment and one that is available at any pharmacy without a prescription. Furthermore, as is the case with nearly any medication, taking the same dose of an opioid antagonist every day produces no more effect than achieving a basic, normal level of biological and personal functioning, becoming "no more impairing than Prozac."[33] The comparison here to a psychoactive medication, an antidepressant, is striking because it is, if one were to fully follow the medical model of addiction, the logical conclusion to draw. If addiction is as much of a brain disease as clinical depression is now seen as (produced by, among other factors, differing levels of neurotransmitters like serotonin), then why shouldn't it be treated medically in much the same way? I would argue that the underlying objections to medical maintenance treatment for addiction rest not on the use of medications, nor on the presence or absence of any particular substance, but because of the way that such treatments condone and normalize the time of addiction and the physical dependence that time has produced. Medical maintenance treatment is a daily practice, extended for an undetermined period of time, that enables the ongoing production of a life; addiction is a daily practice, extended for an undetermined period of time, that enables the production of a life (though not necessarily an ongoing one). The difference, of course, is that medical mainte-

32 Bourgois and Schonberg, *Righteous Dopefiend,* 593.
33 Szalavitz, "How America Overdosed on Drug Courts."

nance treatment enables the production of a more normal life, in which a person is able to hold a job or care for a family outside of the cycle of highs and withdrawals, arrest, and crime of an active addiction. Medical maintenance treatment enables citizenship. Medical maintenance treatment is a material proximity that produces citizenship and access to freedom. Within drug courts, a person's citizenship and future access to citizenship is dependent upon performance within normative, redemptive, and ultimately ideological, non-medical views of treatment and recovery; in maintenance medication treatment, a person's citizenship is dependent upon themselves. While there is certainly a huge amount of work, of "maintenance," to be done, this is ultimately no different from the ideal citizenship that anyone has access to. Medical maintenance treatment accepts the fact of addiction and does not make citizenship and access to freedom dependent upon biology. One of the only ways to avoid the practices of morally-inscribed biological determinism that structured previous epidemics, like that of AIDS, will be to recognize and attend to the very presence of these moral judgments and the biological effects they produce. Making medical treatment available on the basis of moral judgments is far from evidence-based; it is unethical. And ultimately, it will kill as many people as AIDS did before treatment was made available. While we may not be able to know how this epidemic will be historicized, we can at the very least recognize and call out these practices for what they are, now. The opioid epidemic is what it will be.

3

Substance

Risk

The opioid epidemic is many people in deep proximity to the substance of opioids, within the rubrics of addiction and pain treatment, physical dependence and psychological dependence, pain and desire. What is it that maintains any of these proximities, and that keeps people and substances within certain distances? What is it, really, that maintains distances when it comes to any substance? It is a combination of factors and events: architecture, a relationship between the built environment and the legal system, business interests and lobbying groups, personal preferences, human biology, and so on. When it comes to specific substances, and mostly harmful substances, these factors coalesce within the field of risk management. When substances are risky, certain factors and distances take precedence over others, like the legal system and complete removal or abatement of substances like lead or asbestos — an extreme distancing that must always be maintained; there can be little to no safe proximity in relation to such substances. But are these factors and systems adequate when accounting for the proximities of opioids? Do the paradigms of risk management truly answer the question of how one lives with opioids? Given many of the questions and points of contention surrounding opioid use currently, it would seem as if yes, in fact, risk management should be the main guiding discipline. For instance, in questions of who should be given legal access to opioids (who should be exposed or where the risk should be), risk management guidelines may prescribe that only those patients in acute, intractable pain as part of an end-stage terminal disease should be prescribed opioids, thus limiting both the length of an exposure to opioids and relying on the extenuating circumstances of severe pain and end-of-life experiences to counteract, or cancel out, the risks of addiction that opioids pose. But such black and white situations must be extrapolated from, because such extremes are far from the only kind of situation in which opioids are present. Are guidelines like these actually useful when applied to a situation of existing widespread opioid use? Here is where opioids fail to adhere to the models of risk management. With a substance like, again, lead or asbestos, it is not just that the risks of exposure to them are clear, it's that the risks are constant and universal. Asbestos causes mesothelioma in all humans, and lead poisoning will always occur if lead is ingested.

But when it comes to opioids, there has always been an undercurrent of confusions, false appearances, and surprise, an affective structure that undermines the usefulness of risk management in thinking about how to live with opioids. Beginning even with the narratives of surprise within opioid epidemic coverage, and the surprise that these are the people who are dying, opioids have often been (or been representative of) something other than what they seemed to be. And how do you assess the risks and benefits of a substance when what is uncertain lies in the very nature of that substance? Risk management does, of course, deal in uncertainties — but these are often the uncertainties of a future, of what *might* happen. In a proximity to opioids, we encounter uncertainty not within the temporality of opioids but within its very substance. A substantial uncertainty.

Counterfeit

Over the course of the past two years, there has been an incredible surge seen in the rates of overdoses caused by synthetic, incredibly strong opioids. As discussed previously, these substances are most commonly fentanyl and carfentanil, and are usually manufactured in foreign labs and imported, relatively easily and freely, into the United States. Once here, these raw materials are processed in specific yet simple machinery (similarly available for order online) into pill form. These pills are identical in appearance to a pill one would be prescribed. And, in fact, this appearance is intentional, beyond being the appearance of just any opioid pill: drug traffickers and manufacturers commonly manufacture synthetic opioid pills that look identical to OxyContin or Vicodin — pills that command a higher street price than any unlabeled, unknown, synthetic opioid pill would.

Counterfeit pills are an object into which all of the undercurrents of surprise and false appearances within the opioid epidemic have condensed. Counterfeit pills represent the instance, incidence, and accident of dying because you do not know what something really is. Counterfeit pills, as a copy, a substance, and a cause of death, both are and are not unique. On the one hand, counterfeit pills are only able to remain deeply unidentifiable because they take advantage of the very features of "actual" pills that made pills desirable and necessary in the first place: pills were originally manufactured at a point within the history of chemistry and the pharmaceutical industry that marked a turn from plant-based, accessible, small-batch remedies to manufactured and synthetic ones. Pills were manufactured precisely because they provided identical, regular, and assured doses of a substance, *through the very state of uniformity*. Counterfeit pills are a perverse reversal, or deep undermining, of this. On the other hand, the dramatic rise of deaths attributed to counterfeit pills, with deaths due to synthetic opioids alone rising 73% in 2015, stands in unique contrast to anything that has come before it.[1]

1   Associated Press, "A Grim Tally Soars: More than 50,000 Overdose Deaths in US," *STAT,* December 9, 2016, https://www.statnews.com/2016/12/09/opoid-overdose-deaths-us/.

Counterfeit pills are and are not opioid painkillers. In a particularly sick sense, counterfeit pills can be seen as part and parcel of the *you won't believe it's not* industry that has primed consumers to always already be prepared for and desire a product or object that seems like one thing but is actually another. But no one is prepared for this.

To better understand the standing of counterfeit pills and their implications within the opioid epidemic, I will turn to a seminal text concerning authenticity, originality, copies, and aura: Walter Benjamin's "The Work of Art in the Age of Mechanical Reproduction." While this text may be specific to visual art and media, it remains one of the best examinations of the quality or set of qualities a given object has in direct relation to that object's status as original or copy.

The original itself would be the best place to start: "The presence of the original is the prerequisite to the concept of authenticity."[2] And it is this authenticity that does or does not continue through the multiple iterations of copies that surround or are subsequent to an original. It is opioid painkillers that lend a sense of authenticity to counterfeit pills. But what quality, exactly, of painkillers provides this sense of authenticity? While Benjamin may have been referring here to processes of original artworks, like paintings, being reproduced through mechanical techniques, like photography, or theater into film, the relationship Benjamin articulates between originality and authenticity makes clear that what we need to think about here is what is original, *what is necessary*, to have led to the creation of counterfeit pills. With the counterfeit pills, the original is not opioid painkillers per se, but what painkillers are representative of. The original is the feeling of a painkiller. Thus what counterfeit pills reproduce is not an object as such, but *a relation to an object*. Counterfeit pills produce the feeling of being in proximity to opioid painkillers, and the desire and anticipated pleasure and necessity of this proximity. It would also follow that without this

2   Walter Benjamin, "The Work of Art in the Age of Mechanical Reproduction," in *Illuminations: Essays and Reflections,* ed. Hannah Arendt, trans. Harry Zohn (New York: Schocken Books, 1968), 217–52, at 220.

experience of an original, or original experience, a person would not be actively seeking substitutes to that original, when opioid painkillers become out of reach (financially, geographically, or otherwise as shaped by market pressures). And it is these very market pressures that contribute further layers of authenticity to counterfeit pills: it is not only that counterfeit pills are opioid painkillers, but can be the specific objects of OxyContin or Vicodin, the two most widely abused substances within the opioid epidemic and those with the highest street prices.

And yet, counterfeit pills are distinctly not OxyContin nor Vicodin. They are more than either of these substances. This substantiality, the more-ness of counterfeit pills, is a product of exactly the processes of reproduction and mass production they are part of, because "process reproduction can bring out those aspects of the original that are unattainable to the naked eye yet accessible to the lens…can capture images which escape natural vision…technical reproduction can put the copy of the original into situations which would be out of reach for the original itself."[3] Counterfeit pills are an object in which the substance of opioids is able to inhabit and occupy different situations, spaces, and proximities than "original" or "actual" pills do. Counterfeit pills can, for instance, kill a person at rates and at a speed out of reach for more common, legally manufactured forms of opioids. Particularly at the level of a single pill: a single pill made of carfentanil or fentanyl can and does act in ways drastically different from an identical looking pill made of morphine or oxycodone; a lethal dose of fentanyl is 2 mg, approximately the size of a grain of salt.[4] It is not just the fact of reproduction, but the illicit or black market nature of this reproduction that positions counterfeit pills in this way; what makes counterfeit pills deadly is a change in substance, in nature, without a change in form. Does this mean that the groups of people manufacturing and distributing counterfeit pills are intentionally trying to kill

3   Benjamin, "The Work of Art," 220.
4   US Department of Justice, Drug Enforcement Administration, "Fentanyl: A Briefing Guide for First Responders," June 2017, https://www.dea.gov/druginfo/Fentanyl_BriefingGuideforFirstResponders_June2017.pdf.

people? No. It means, more so, that market pressures, the market pressures that drive the desirability for massively available forms of opioids, are also bodily pressures and deadly pressures. The opioid epidemic is many people in the same place at the same time and the pressure of this mass.

Within this situation surrounding counterfeit pills, we can see the ways that a desire for an original (including, especially, an original feeling) outweighs or interacts with the unique capabilities of a copy. In other words, intense, addictive desires tied to an original experience outweigh what is also common knowledge of the dangers of opioids, particularly among active drug users who may have witnessed or have first hand knowledge of the overdose of another. At what point, if any, does this transform into or become a desire for the copy itself? At the point, perhaps, of an epidemic. Benjamin identifies this point or movement as what happens when "making many reproductions…substitutes a plurality of copies for a unique existence."[5] This speaks to the very nature of an epidemic of drug abuse, especially when seen in relation to the patterns of drug manufacture and trafficking counterfeit pills are a part of; this speaks to the very nature of the mass market, of mass desire and pain, of the many qualities of many bodies in the same place and the qualities and shapes of the many desires of those bodies. Furthermore, the details of the manufacture of counterfeit pills provides a more pragmatic reading of Benjamin's sentiment. Attempting to stay one step ahead of US law enforcement, as newer synthetic substances become identified and banned, overseas labs manufacture endless variations of similar chemicals in order to sustain and guarantee a stable, easily distributed supply. The plurality of substances is far more important than any's unique existence.

Beyond sheer mass, what drives a desire for a copy, or what enables a desire to become detached from an original and move towards a copy? In a sense, this is the very nature of addiction. As Benjamin notes in relation to the desires at the heart of processes of reproduction: "Every day the urge grows stronger to get hold of an object at very close range by way of its likeness, its

5   Benjamin, "The Work of Art," 221.

reproduction."[6] In a moment of desperation and withdrawal, what matters is the closeness and immediacy of an opioid — not necessarily precisely which opioid it is, especially if you cannot ever identify it until after the fact. Desire is inseparable from time and distance, from proximity, and the feeling of such a distance over time, especially in relation to opioid addiction, and the state of having been in this proximity for longer periods of time. As a deeply cyclical disease and a disease of habits, addiction imparts deeper layers to an understanding of the idea that "the unique value of the 'authentic' work of art has its basis in ritual."[7] Taking a pill, the feeling of taking a pill, the feelings after taking a pill, are both unique values and rituals in which an addiction may originate, and simultaneously the very state that allows certain desires tied to an original to become unhinged. What is authentic and original can be overtaken, canceled out. Every high is exactly like the one before it, and nothing like the one before it. Habit, as much as it is about sameness, is also always the medium of the most drastic changes. In illustration, I would point to the nature and use of a recent pharmaceutical development within the opioid epidemic. In attempts to maintain access to opioid painkillers for those patients who need them (and maintain wide profit margins on newer, patented, and non-generic opioid forms), the pharmaceutical industry has been widely touting the benefits of newly developed ADFs, abuse deterrent formulations. These pills, in a sense, attempt to be identical to opioid painkillers in every effect if not in every quality, in that they provide as effective pain relief, but cannot be crushed or otherwise tampered with in ways drug abusers may utilize. Yet these pills fail to be convincing or successful in preventing drug abuse, as "drug abusers quickly drop the reformulated drugs in favor of older painkillers or heroin."[8] The object of the pill no longer matters: the originality of an experience with "older painkillers or heroin"

6   Benjamin, "The Work of Art," 223.
7   Benjamin, "The Work of Art," 224.
8   Associated Press and the Center for Public Integrity, "Drug Makers Push a Profitable but Unproven Opioid Solution," *STAT,* December 15, 2016, https://www.statnews.com/2016/12/15/drugmakers-unproven-opioid-solution/.

becomes stronger and more desirable than any other, even non-counterfeit, opioid experience.

Counterfeit pills are a point within what is really a constellation of physical, social, and political diseases, situations, and affects that these undercurrents of originality, desire, and copies are moving through. From poverty and the daily small violence of the rural to HIV, hepatitis C and other illnesses related to intravenous drug use, people engaged in and encountering one of these instances, like counterfeit pills, are far more likely to be simultaneously or soon thereafter entangled in a related instance. Drawing on the work of anthropologist Merrill Singer, these clusters of illnesses that "[encompass] nonbiological conditions like poverty…and other social, economic and political factors known to accompany poor health,"[9] can be termed *syndemics*. One could, therefore, detail a syndemic of opioid use within the United States as existing as or within a cluster including: both licit and illicit pharmaceutical manufacturing, poverty, joblessness, global drug policy, lack of social support, addiction and substance abuse, diseases related to IV drug use, overdoses, opioid withdrawal, and so forth. Studying the patterns of physical illness and social situations of a heroin-using population in Hartford, CT, Singer termed the cluster he found to be a *syringe-mediated syndemic*.[10] Given the prevalence of not only counterfeit pills, but pills generally, I would argue that the opioid epidemic is *pill-mediated*: pills are the technology that is both actively being used to transport, distribute, and ingest the substance of opioids, and this specific technology, whether intentionally or not, is providing the parameters within which these actions — and their consequences — are taking place. Pills are easy to distribute, easy to take, and easy to produce large quantities of. They require no paraphernalia to abuse, though some users do crush or otherwise augment them to make pills injectable or able to be snorted or smoked. As users transition to drugs like heroin or otherwise begin using intravenous methods,

9   Jessica Wapner, "Austin, Indiana: The HIV Capital of Small-town America," *Mosiac,* May 2, 2016, https://mosaicscience.com/story/austin-indiana-hiv-america-syndemics.
10 Wapner, "Austin, Indiana."

rates of related diseases will rise (and have been), though as the opioid epidemic has focused on pills, this has been much less of an epidemic of diseases like HIV or hepatitis than it could have been. Though easily manufactured, pills (particularly legal, branded forms like OxyContin) fetch high street prices; driving a transition to heroin is often the fact that heroin is less expensive than pills. Even within a brief sketch of the current situation as a pill-mediated syndemic, we can see the breadth of causal factors and effects, from economic to biological, that are generated by qualities of the pills themselves. "Epidemic," while still a useful word for its sheer mass, may also not be entirely what it seems, or encompass all there is.

For the people who are dying, of either counterfeit or "actual" pills, how do these layers of false appearances affect their deaths? Though this practice has begun to change, it was common during many of the early years of the opioid epidemic for death certificates to not list "overdose" or "substance abuse" as a cause of death; acute intoxication or respiratory failure or an otherwise accidental and unspecified instance were more commonly used.[11] As the consequences of this practice have become apparent (primarily pertaining to the miscollection of opioid use and overdose statistics it engenders) and it has begun to be discontinued, such death certificates still present another instance of false appearances within the opioid epidemic: a statistical false appearance, or the false appearance (or presentation) of many deaths. What is it about an addiction that disqualifies it as a cause of death, aside from stigma? If one were to fully follow a model in which addiction is a disease, would it not make sense to consider an overdose as part of the prognosis? With the rates of overdose and death for opioid addicts so high, such a conceptualization is not unfounded; the data certainly supports the fact that overdoses are a frequent end of addiction. And thinking of an overdose death in this way would make it more analogous to experiences with death in other diseases. While an infection may not be

---

11 Jeff Cohen, "Details On Death Certificates Offer Layers Of Clues To Opioid Epidemic," *National Public Radio,* June 1, 2016, http://www. npr.org/sections/health-shots/2016/06/01/479440834/in-opioid-crisis-it-s-important-to-know-which-drugs-caused-a-death.

completely expected as a cause of death in cancer, it is absolutely understood to be a normal event for a terminal cancer patient. But even while drawing this comparison, it is possible to recognize the paradoxical situation at the heart of how an overdose is perceived and talked about: how can something feel so inevitable, yet always be so surprising?

Over the course of the epidemic as a whole, it becomes apparent that time itself is frequently what creates this disjuncture between inevitability and surprise, contributing to an overall sense of disbelief. Epidemics, as a function of epidemiology, are always already about and structured by time, through many instances happening at the same time — and by the fact that the collection and interpretation of epidemiological statistical data takes time. Often, it seems, it is the slowness of this process — particularly as interpretations become translated into policies and public health recommendations — that directly contributes to a sense of things not being what they seem. Perhaps it would be more accurate to say that things do not anymore seem like what they once were. One of the clearest instances of this process and its consequences can be found in recent data collected for the state of Massachusetts. Struggling with some of the highest rates of opioid abuse in the nation, both state and local governments have been active in working to bring down not only abuse but prescribing rates. And, in fact, they have been successful in these efforts: opioid prescribing rates for Massachusetts have decreased in 2016 from previous levels. However, overdose death rates are on track to make 2016 the deadliest year yet[12]. There are and are not clear answers to explain this pattern. On the one hand, it could be assumed that a vast majority of overdose deaths are being caused by stronger synthetic substances, and the data certainly shows a rise in availability of and overdoses due to synthetic opioids. On the other hand, it continues to be true that prescription pills, including nonopioids like benzodiazepines,

12 Martha Bebinger, "Roughly 5 Mass. Residents Are Dying Daily Due to Overdose, Most Involving Fentanyl," *CommonHealth* (blog), *WBUR*, November 7, 2016, http://www.wbur.org/commonhealth/2016/11/07/overdose-deaths-fentanyl.

continue to be found in significant numbers of overdoses.[13] Is this simply a legislative false appearance? What, exactly, is out of sync? How long does something have to seem like one thing, like what it is, in order to actually be that thing?

Sackler

This last question, in particular, applies as much to pain patients as to anyone else involved in the opioid epidemic. How long does opioid use have to continue for it to no longer seem like medication, but physical dependence? How long does a person have to be in pain, or how much pain, to outweigh what seem like risks? At what point does a pain patient themselves come to seem like a different kind of person as shaped by beliefs about their substance use? Just as any opioid user is acting in an environment that has become deeply saturated with these substances, so too are pain patients, and in ways that may be even more imperceptible: the status of a pain patient in recovery from prior substance abuse issues may be paradigmatic of this sentiment.

Though this could also be illustrated with a much more personal example. I, myself, seem like any other pain patient (despite not having any of the most common conditions, like back pain or arthritis, that opioids are frequently prescribed for) and I am like any other pain patient, but this status is not constant. Like any relationship, my proximity to opioids is shaped by the physical space I find myself in. One of the most complex, opioid-saturated spaces that I find myself in frequently and, at times, even daily, is that of Harvard Square. Upon entering this space, many other instances and situations become apparent within the frame of "pain patient" than may meet the eye initially.

13 See Felice J. Freyer, "Overdose Deaths in Mass. Continue to Surge," *The Boston Globe,* November 7, 2016, https://www.bostonglobe.com/metro/2016/11/07/overdose-deaths-mass-continue-surge/z9AdKhXF-43NAhngHYvTguO/story.html, and Massachusetts Department of Public Health, "Data Brief: Opioid-related Overdose Deaths Among Massachusetts Residents," August 2016, http://www.mass.gov/eohhs/docs/dph/quality/drugcontrol/county-level-pmp/opioid-related-overdose-deaths-among-ma-residents-august-2016.pdf.

This happens because of the proximity of bodies. There is, on the northeast edge of Harvard Square, the presence of Arthur M. Sackler. A founder and CEO of Purdue Pharma, along with his brother, Sackler has become known as the father of modern medical advertising. Through his positions within the pharmaceutical industry and as an owner of an advertising agency, Sackler developed the techniques like direct-to-doctor advertising that have subsequently become the mainstay of pharmaceutical marketing, and were put to particular use in the aggressive marketing of OxyContin.[14] Though he passed away in the early 1990s, Sackler remains in the square through his endowment of the Sackler Museum of Art at Harvard University.[15] OxyContin can be found, in a sense, throughout the rest of Harvard Square as well. Long home to groups of homeless or itinerant individuals, Harvard Square is often a space in which people are more or less visibly using drugs in public; the majority of experiences I've had in witnessing people unconscious or nodding off in public have happened in and around Harvard Square. While it is difficult to ascertain how many people are using opioids there at any given time, Middlesex County, of which the city of Cambridge and thus Harvard Square are a part, have had the highest number of opioid deaths over the past 15 years in the state, and Middlesex County continues to have the highest rate of opioid abuse in Massachusetts.[16]

14 See Sam Quinones, *Dreamland: The True Tale of America's Opiate Epidemic* (London: Bloomsbury, 2015).
15 The Sacklers, whether Arthur, Raymond, or Mortimer, also inhabit via endowment substantial spaces at the Metropolitan Museum of Art (where the Sackler Wing houses the Temple of Dendur), Tufts University, the Smithsonian, and the Ashmolean. For a comprehensive overview of their philanthropy and business practices, see Christopher Glazek, "The Secretive Family Making Billions From The Opioid Crisis," *Esquire,* October 16, 2017, https://www.esquire.com/news-politics/a12775932/sackler-family-oxycontin/, and Patrick Radden Keefe, "The Family that Built an Empire of Pain," *The New Yorker,* October 30, 2017, https://www.newyorker.com/magazine/2017/10/30/the-family-that-built-an-empire-of-pain.
16 Massachusetts Department of Public Health, "Number of Unintentional Opioid-Related Overdose Deaths by County, MA

I am exactly where one of these things ends and the other begins. I have, at times, been dependent on Harvard University, either as an employee or because of the employment of my partner; I have also been tied to the museum itself through my position as an editor at an arts-focused publication, and have attended events and exhibitions there as the museum's guest. It is difficult to determine how directly I have benefitted from the money of Sackler, or of the museum, but however roundabout this may be, it is present. Though I have only been prescribed OxyContin once, during an emergency room visit, I have paid for other opioid prescriptions with money more or less tied to Harvard; this relationship is almost cyclical. On the other hand, I am deeply, biologically, in proximity to all those within the square abusing or using opioids: opioids are *ours*—even as the legislation of opioids and the experience of that legislation has come to belong very much more to some people than to others. This relationship, for me, has become condensed within a particular set of objects within the square, a set of public restroom stalls. The First Church, located near the northern side of the square, has maintained public restrooms throughout its lengthy history, but closed these restrooms in 2012 as the church administration no longer felt they were able to handle the opioid overdoses that were or might take place there. Following this closure, local business owners saw a sudden rise in people using their front steps or back alleys as restrooms. The Harvard Square Business Association, a lobbying group that has also recently played a major role in other urban planning and redevelopment decisions in the area, participated in a lobbying effort to have the city of Cambridge install public restrooms to replace those closed by the First Church. The city did so, and spent $400,000 to install the two, now operational, stalls.[17] On every walk

Residents: 2000–2015," November 2016, http://www.mass.gov/ eohhs/docs/dph/stop-addiction/current-statistics/overdose-deaths-by- county-nov-2016.pdf.

17 See Steve Annear, "Cambridge to Open City's First Freestanding Outdoor Public Toilet," *The Boston Globe,* February 8, 2016, https:// www.bostonglobe.com/metro/2016/02/08/cambridge-open-city-first- freestanding-outdoor-public-toilet/WKAELRk7GpLPSUZg7xLCYI/

through Harvard Square, now, I think about the money of these restrooms: who was it spent for? How many doses of naloxone, the overdose reversal medication, could this have paid for? What does this money, used in this way, express? I think, too, of all of the overdose awareness posters on all of the trash cans throughout Boston: because of their solar compacting ability and design, each of these trash cans costs $2,000; $2,000 plastered with the outstretched hands of presumed "junkies," but not, directly, money supporting such people.

These instances of the legal-architectural relations contained within or engendered by opioids are and are not uniquely current. Boston, in particular, has long been shaped by the money of opioids. On university buildings and hospitals throughout the city, one can see the names of families whose money was made in 18th- and 19th-century import-export businesses, primarily focused on the distribution of opium in China: Perkins, Cabot, Cushing, and Delano. Perkins, in particular, was influential in the founding of Massachusetts General Hospital, McLean Hospital, and the Perkins School for the Blind.[18] Elsewhere throughout the city, one can visit the Cabot Library at Harvard or the Cabot Intercultural Center at Tufts (or the Sackler School of Graduate Biomedical Sciences, also at Tufts).

If nothing else, it is illustrative of the many objects of opioids, beyond what is apparent. While opioids are, of course, painkillers and pills, they are also: money, specific buildings and the names on those buildings, institutions (and institutionalized), lines written into city budgets, objects encountered in public areas. What this situation and space demonstrates is the way that a material proximity, as in my own personal proximity as it is augmented by my presence and embeddedness within this (public, institutional) space, is a *legal-architectural relationship.*

story.html, and Katharine Q. Seelye, "Heroin Epidemic Increasingly Seeps Into Public View, *The New York Times,* March 6, 2016, https://www.nytimes.com/2016/03/07/us/heroin-epidemic-increasingly-seeps-into-public-view.html.

18 Bebinger, "How Profits From Opium Shaped 19th-Century Boston," *CommonHealth* (blog), *WBUR,* July 31, 2017, http://www.wbur.org/commonhealth/2017/07/31/opium-boston-history.

It is produced from interactions between physical and legal bodies, and from the way that the written law structures the built environment (as in, for the most obvious example, building codes). It is not constant. It is always, simultaneously social, biological, economic, and political. It is the way I walk past groups of other opioid users, and the stack of pay stubs I have from Harvard University; it is the budget and policies passed by the city of Cambridge, and it is the press releases I receive from the museum. It is my own pain, and the physical, emotional, and economic pain of those within the square who are also using, if differently, opioids. It is a relationship of multiples. What does it take to notice beyond false appearances, beyond what is simply a name on a building or a person on a sidewalk? What does it take to notice how much opioids contain?

Using

Through all of these instances of false appearances and mimesis, opioids disrupt the norms set by the histories of other dangerous (and useful) substances within the disciplines of risk management and public health. Opioids are neither something to be entirely avoided, never used again (as if that were even possible, now, given the presence of illicit labs manufacturing synthetic forms of these drugs) nor a substance that should (continue to) be prescribed widely — nor even, always, a substance that is visible and apparent enough to be avoided. Opioids are a gray area. Because of these disciplinary disruptions, a relationship and proximity to opioids also exists in and as a disruption to normal and existing ideas about how we understand a substance to act within our bodies.

A normal idea of how a harmful, perhaps addiction-causing substance acts within our bodies is set by the paradigms of risk management and, I would argue, fields of ecology epitomized by studies like Rachel Carson's *Silent Spring*, which examined the effects of a chemical or outright toxic substance within an ecosystem:[19] a harmful substance produces the effects it does because of an exposure to *too much*; whether through repetition

19 Rachel Carson, *Silent Spring* (Boston, MA: Houghton Mifflin, 1962).

over time or a sheer initial quantity, a harmful substance over-whelms the body of the organism or ecosystem it is released into, wreaking havoc because it throws what had been there out of balance. Within our own bodies, the most basic model we have that conceptualizes this harmful substance-balanced ecosystem (or substance-self) relationship is that of eating. This is a model based on putting something in sensibly, having sensible and insensible or invisible things happen to it, and having both sensible and insensible or invisible (inasmuch as they are much slower things) come out or become apparent. The indicators we have for what a substance, like food, is doing to or within us exists on a wide spectrum of times and timing, encompassing both slow-to-immediate and singular-to-repetitive: weight gain, allergic reactions, feeling more energetic, feeling tired, having a headache, having cravings. How long does something have to seem like a thing in order to be that thing?

Another way to express this substance-self relationship and our experience of it would be through a neuroscientific lens and an explanation of the somatosensory system and the somesthetic senses it produces. To apprehend and understand an object, whether an internal body part or state or an external object, the body and nervous system continually, minutely, and across multiple body areas and systems collects data: signals that travel within the nervous system to the brain, becoming neural pat-terns that generate actions, whether the regulation of hormones within the bloodstream or a set of emotional responses and the physiological states that accompany them (i.e., the involvement of the hormone cortisol in the affective and physical "fight or flight response"). The importance of the somatosensory system in this process is twofold. First, by constantly monitoring bodily signals, homeostasis is simultaneously monitored and regu-lated: incoming signals about too much or too little of a given hormone, say, will prompt the brain to send signals that correct any imbalance. Secondly, the importance of bodily signals and the body maps they produce is crucial within an understand-ing of consciousness, of knowing awareness, as consisting of "constructing knowledge about two facts: that the organism is involved in relating to some object, and that the object in the relation is causing a change in the organism."[20] In other words, in order to understand how a substance acts within our bodies, we must be able to *both* gather information about the substance and information about ourselves; ultimately, information about our proximities.

Thus, to understand an object, we rely on primary sensory systems (i.e. visual, auditory, touch) to record different aspects of an object, and integrate them to produce an experience of the object. For instance, I am relying on my sense of touch to record the softness of this particular sofa, which I will recall later when choosing a seat. Crucially, it is not only sensory data that is recorded and remembered, but the response we had to that object (which is always simultaneously emotional and physiological, consisting of "feelings" and mechanical, thermal, and chemical reactions that accompany them), thereby producing perception and recall. When we remember an object, we always also remember how it *felt*, even when those feelings may appear to be just a series of nonconscious motor adjustments made in the presence of the object. What this should recall is our discussion of the necessity of an emotional experience of an original opioid in subsequently producing a desire for even a copy of an opioid, an instance in which clearly what is being recalled is both the object of the pill and the feeling of taking a pill — and the clear effects of this kind of emotional and biological recollection. How we understand a substance is thus always based on physical aspects of the substance itself (the size and shape and weight of a pill) and our physical and emotional reaction *within an encounter with that substance* (how good it felt to take a pill; how this desire may extend to similar, even if crucially different, objects of the same size and shape and weight). Here, therefore, we may expand our understanding of a material proximity to include even more deeply the biological and emotional, and the constant interplay and inseparability of the two. A material proximity describes the way that a relationship to an object, down to the level of nonconscious, nervous system workings, is always generated both by characteristics of the object and characteristics of ourselves.

20 Antonio Damasio, *The Feeling of What Happens: Body and Emotion in the Making of Consciousness* (New York: Harcourt Brace, 1999), 135.

This complex process involving multiple physiological systems, only a portion of which we may have conscious access to at any given moment is, in a way, a kind of behind-the-scenes orchestration of our bodies and actions — all, ultimately, in the aim of maintaining homeostasis, to return to the former noted importance of the somatosensory system. The practice of maintaining steady, precisely calibrated levels and rates of *everything* within a body, from blood oxygen levels to insulin production, homeostasis is the basis of life and its maintenance. This is not to say that the levels maintained by homeostasis will be permanent and unchanging within the life of a given individual. As we saw in the neuroscience of addiction, long-term alteration of homeostatic levels (such as, within addiction to opioids, levels of dopamine and other neurotransmitters) leads to a state referred to as *allostasis*: given the elasticity of the nervous system, in particular, homeostatic processes can be altered and then, in a way, reset and maintained at these new, altered levels. The amount of change a body can withstand and maintain is termed the allostatic load.[21] Simultaneously, of course, elasticity is not the same thing as positive change; as "load" would suggest, allostasis takes a toll on the body that sustains it, physiologically and emotionally, as in the case of addiction. And this is where the field of ecology and its substance-ecosystem conceptualizations become especially relevant and equivocal to the way we conceptualize a substance within a body, whether through the terminology of allostasis and homestasis, the model of eating (and weight gain or weight loss) or the social constructs of "once an addict, always an addict" — a proximity to any substance can potentially *overwhelm* because of the ability of a substance to throw off the normal functioning (homeostasis) of a body or group of bodies (an epidemic). What is of crucial importance to the way that this relationship is expressed about opioids or other addicting substances is that at the very center of the model is the black box of the body: while we may know what we put in and (eventually) what comes out, and while our somatosensory system may translate mechanical, chemical, or thermal data into feelings and behaviors, we do not

---

21 Markus Heilig, *The Thirteenth Step: Addiction in the Age of Brain Science* (New York: Columbia University Press, 2015), 84.

consciously know what is going on "in between." What becomes overwhelming cannot, always or reliably, be predicted, nor is it always true that just because a substance was not overwhelming before means that it will not be overwhelming next time, especially given that we are always also constructing an experience of and knowledge about a substance based on prior personal experience. While "it is a biological error to confuse what a person puts in their mouth with what it becomes after it is swallowed," it is one of the most common and accepted errors.[22] And one that becomes even more common and acceptable when surrounding it are layers of sociocultural constructs that surround substance-individual relationships involved in addiction, or other common conditions like obesity, in which an obese person is equated with the "bad fat" they must surely be consuming, thereby mistaking not only what a person puts in their mouth with what it becomes after it is swallowed, but what a person puts in their mouth with who *they* become. You are what you eat.

What bridges this conceptual transition from ideas about a substance (bad fat) to ideas about a person (bad fat person) are a series of categories used to classify substances, which incorporate and are based on physical, somatosensory information about an object, personal and emotional experiences of an object, a recollection of these experiences, information about others' physical and emotional experiences, and, again, our own emotional and physical relationships to this information. In other words, substance categorization is both scientific, as in based on the collection and interpretation of physical data, and a sociocultural construct, as in based on the collection and interpretation of ideas about other people. Used to describe the risks, benefits, and uses of both sensible and insensible proximities to substances, these categories include: carcinogen, medicine, placebo, vitamin, nutrient, healthy, fat, and so on, with many subcategories and related instances therein, like that of cure with the category of medicine, or carcinogen and fat existing within a broader category that may be termed either toxic or harmful. The category

22 Ian Leslie, "The Sugar Conspiracy," *The Guardian,* April 7, 2016, https://www.theguardian.com/society/2016/apr/07/the-sugar-conspiracy-robert-lustig-john-yudkin.

we believe a substance exists in drives our behaviors in the use or avoidance of that substance. As much as possible, we try to avoid carcinogens, based on scientific data collected about the physical effects of certain substances and our emotional responses given the experience of people subjected to these effects; nutrients we try to eat as much of as possible, difficult as it may be to identify how much of one we may be getting, given scientific data that informs current nutritional recommendations and sociocultural premiums placed on healthy eating and/as thinness. Thus, though these categories are in no way unchanging or uninfluenced by the science and culture of the time, substance categorization does drive black and white thinking about proximities to substances. Within this model, substances become objects to avoid or incorporate; everything is either good or bad, or pain or relief. And while there are certainly examples of substances that change from one category to the next (as in the recent revision of fat from a "purely" bad substance to a healthy or beneficial one, at least in certain forms) there are less examples of substances that exist simultaneously in multiple categories, or that fully express the transitoriness or multiplicity of the category they are situated in. Except, perhaps, for very specific substances within the category of drugs used in medicine, which may provide both beneficial, even pleasurable effects and simultaneously negative effects — but even here, we have a category to separate these effects, overriding a conceptualization of the multiplicity of a substance: side effects.

And it is in this last category, of course, where we may find opioids, providing both relief and pain. Exemplified by the very term *painkiller*, as if a double negative, *pain + killer,* always produces a positive. It is the many double negatives of opioids that prove so disruptive to ideas about substance use as shaped by substance categorization. Opioids *do* kill people, and are, in fact, killing many people; opioids *do* treat pain effectively, and there are very few other effective options for the treatment of intractable pain. How should opioids be categorized? How do we understand — and come to accept, incorporate, and work around — the limits of category-based conceptualizations? What can be abated? What can be maintained?

Living With

When we find ourselves in proximity to opioids, when we are living with opioids as pain patients or as someone abusing drugs, and when this proximity is taking place within a sociocultural context in which substance-related behaviors are shaped by processes of categorizing substances, themselves based on physical, emotional, and neurological experiences, what assumptions and ideas predicated on the substance are we with — and how do we choose to act, based on the multiplicity of these ideas? How do you live with opioids? How, when conceptualizing a proximity to opioids as a substance-ecosystem relationship, do you maintain balance?

Ultimately, these questions are about the affective and physical *work of managing relations to substances*. Not unlike other homeostatic processes, we do this work continually, making minute adjustments and reevaluating our proximities constantly. The difference, though, when acting around and with substances that produce affective and emotional experiences is that this work can never be completely physical, as if injecting heroin to return to a high is just like regulating levels of blood sugar. This affective work of managing relations to substances, while perhaps extreme in the case of heroin, is actually incredibly common and simple: just think of how many people, across so many substances, regulate their proximity to a substance based on the perceived or known effects of that substance set against time and within an emotional field in order to generate limitations and guidelines for their proximity. For instance, the diet plans that set aside two days a week for eating whatever you want after five days of intermittent fasting, or the perceived difference between an occasional after-work drink and daily drinking. Guidelines for substance use like these, whether for a drug like alcohol or an everyday substance like food, are thus time-based, physical parameters (two days a week for eating anything) that become affectively reinforced (if my proximity remains within these parameters, I'll lose weight, maintain health, etc.). It is also important to note that within this affective reinforcement is another layer of what is being managed through our material proximities: it is not just that we manage physical experiences *to* substances, but that we manage our relations to our own emotional states and experiences *through* substances. In other words, it is not just that we choose to regulate our relationship to food as reinforced by affective logic, as in the dieting example, but that we regulate our relationship to our own emotions through food — in other words, the very existence of the term "comfort food."

This work of managing physical experiences through affectively-reinforced logic is based on *the expectation of force and the force of expectation*. While we will return to this concept in a later chapter in much greater detail, for now we can understand this on its most basic level: we expect a substance to produce effects with a given forcefulness, and the force of our expectations becomes the affective structure that reinforces the logic of our use and its parameters. For instance, if we expect a substance (say, a single cookie) to exert relatively little force in producing an expected or known effect when encountered in a given process and performed only once or for a limited time (how eating a single cookie once will not make me gain weight) then we may be much more likely to go ahead and use that substance, or remain in proximity to it. On the other hand, if we expect a substance to exert a powerful force when producing a known or expected effect, and we know that we will be in proximity to that substance repetitively or for a long time (how eating a dozen cookies every day will, most likely, make me gain weight), then we may be more likely not to use that substance.

Of course, what about when we don't know? Within my own proximity to opioids, should I expect pain or relief? Or, is pain relief or the possibility of addiction a stronger force? Is my expectation of pain relief a stronger force than the force of addiction? While we can turn to data collected scientifically to address these questions, as in a recent study that demonstrated that most pain patients are, contrary to the constant media rhetoric that says otherwise, actually unlikely to develop long-term opioid abuse,[23] we also are always effected by personal and emotional

23 Pat Anson, "Few Pain Patients Become Long-Term Opioid Users," *Pain News Network,* January 2, 2017, https://www.painnewsnetwork. org/stories/2017/1/2/few-pain-patients-become-long-term-opioid-

experiences, like my reaction to what I have come to understand about everyone around me being affected by opioids. Are sets of expectations like these — and their forces — always calibrated by fear? And with this fear is there not always also the specter of blame, in the event of failure? In many ways, these questions are more easily answered when we are thinking about how substances act in others' bodies. An ease, perhaps, generated by the fact that in judging others what we have access to is only the visual, or observational (as of their behaviors), and at a slight remove from the intricacies of our own personal affective logics. Again, dieting or obesity and the *you are what you eat* principle make this clear. We understand substances to act within others' bodies as predicated on an assumption of free choice and what a failure to choose "correctly" looks like — i.e., obese people are such because they chose to eat the foods they did, or chose not to exercise, etc. This, of course, completely disregards that which may be beyond the realm of the immediately apparent and perceptible, like genetic predispositions, environmental factors influenced by sociopolitical and economic systems, and so on. The same holds true for opioid abuse, particularly as we have already seen within narrative tropes like that of the standing of addicts as victims/perpetrators. In short, this is the view that "people should be responsible for what they put into their bodies."[24] Given that this quote was taken from a participant in a survey about blame within the opioid epidemic, it is clear that with responsibility always comes (potential) blame; that these questions about the risks and perceptions of the effects of opioids, and how these risks and perceptions should or are already affecting the use of opioids, are not only about who should be at risk, but who produced the risk in the first place and who should be at fault — even when a substance is only producing the effects (binding to *mu* receptors, changing neurotransmitter levels) that it would in *any* person. In the survey quoted, a majority of people blamed doctors for reckless overprescribing, an attitude that

users.

24 Dylan Scott, "1 in 3 Americans Blame Doctors for National Opioid Epidemic, STAT-Harvard Poll Finds," *STAT,* March 17, 2017, https://www.statnews.com/2016/03/17/stat-harvard-opioid-poll/.

can also be seen in countless other instances of opioid epidemic coverage. Even within a scenario in which groups like major companies within the pharmaceutical industry have clearly played a predominant role in producing the opioid epidemic, we are still more likely to place blame on an individual.

This focus perpetuates misunderstandings and ultimately allows for the continuation of, if not the epidemic itself, at least behaviors, systems, and scenarios that have led to it. By focusing on the responsibilities of individuals who we assume are "free" to make choices when encountering a substance and acting in relation to it, even when there is no definitive information available about that substance or whose effects may be unpredictable, we fail to fully attend to the systemic nature of substance-based proximities. Even when this systemic nature can become apparent within our own personal experiences, like the institutional and legal-architectural nature of opioids within my experience of Harvard Square, it remains invisible elsewhere. One may, instead, continue to focus on the groups of opioid-abusing people within the Square or county. The conceptual difficulty in articulating this issue is the slight but ever-present suggestion within these ideas that individuals are entirely not free, that individuals simply, somehow, "happen upon" a substance—an attitude that comes dangerously close to the "people becoming subject to a substance" attitude of a larger addiction rhetoric. This is not what I mean to suggest. It is possible, instead, to maintain a position that allows for a broad multiplicity in understanding the material proximities people come into and maintain. People are free to choose in relation to substances, and many have chosen to take opioids; at the same time, both this initial decision and the subsequent decision(s) to continue taking opioids are shaped in part, yet definitively, by biological and neurological factors that are not within the conscious control of an individual; at the same time, perhaps an individual is aware of these biological factors to begin with, and can choose or try to choose to act accordingly; at the same time, the very fact that so many people have so many opportunities to encounter and choose to act towards opioids is not a neutral fact but a product of governmental and medical-industrial relationships. People being "free" to choose—and thus people being "always" at fault—is in no way constant or singular. A material proximity condenses these factors. And in appearing to be a singular situation, or a singular act of taking opioids, this kind of condensation can make such proximities easier to judge. But no less easy to experience.

To challenge such an attitude focused on individuals and choice one could ask, instead of "how do you live with opioids," a question focused on a mass of individuals: how do you live with the opioid epidemic? In living with an epidemic, one is not only living within an environment saturated with a specific substance, but an environment more generally saturated and overwhelmed. In living with this epidemic and sensing the pressures of it, I feel myself to be living with prior epidemics as well, and their residues — specifically, again, that of the AIDS epidemic. In living with the opioid epidemic now, the residues of the sheer loss of life, medical and governmental inaction, and the physical consequences of social assumptions and attitudes within the AIDS epidemic have come to coat my current experience. In living with this residue, I am living with the immobility of policy or the irreconcilability of policy and daily experiences of pain, in multiple senses, places, and situations. This irreconcilability is apparent in the institutional and legal-architectural nature of opioids far beyond any specific or personal space. For instance, why is it that treatment centers, particularly those focused on medical maintenance treatment, are relatively few and far between and difficult to access? Is this a reflection of the substance itself, something unique to methadone, or a product of governmental systems as influenced by popular opinion? And when it becomes apparent, whether related to residues of the AIDS epidemics or living with opioids, now, that the saturated environment we are to be living with is such because of systemic, legal-architectural relationships like these, should we not understand *substance abuse* to include not only the behaviors of an individual, but exactly this network of governmental, industrial, and medical powers that move, and move through, substances and distribute them? What becomes abusive? What can be accounted for, or held accountable? What is one encountering in proximity to a substance, and what can be taken responsibility for? What can be abated?

4

Pain

Pain

Pain is a thing that happens. Pain patients are people to whom the thing of pain has happened, is happening to, will happen to, or is continuing to happen to. The things of pain patients commonly include low back pain, arthritis, post-surgical pain, and the pain of accidents and injuries. For low back pain, in fact, opioids are the now most commonly prescribed class of drugs.[1] The pain of opioids, addiction, and the pain of what is and is not being called desire is not within this (part of the) epidemic. Also categorically different is the pain of cancer patients and those with other chronic illnesses; I can say that I am a pain patient, but more accurately I am a patient being treated for a pancreatic disease. As much pain as it may cause, my disease is not really itself pain. The pain of pain patients is something else. Something separate, one must assume, from illness as such, as otherwise the thousands of people frequently named pain patients would be referred to

1   Richard A. Deyo, Michael Von Korff, and David Duhrkoop, "Opioids for Low Back Pain," *British Medical Journal* 350 (2015): g6380, https://doi.org/10.1136/bmj.g6380.

instead as patients of specific diseases. Or sick people. It is therefore not such a leap to assume or imagine that pain patients must be otherwise healthy people experiencing pain — whose pain does not alter their fundamental health or their status as able-bodied. It is also not a leap to assume that it was exactly these people whom doctors discovered following the adoption of pain as a fifth vital sign in the 1990s. Neither this change in medical practice nor aggressive pharmaceutical marketing alone fully explain the vast rise in opioid prescribing throughout the 1990s and early 2000s. It could not simply have been that because doctors began looking for and measuring pain that they also began treating it; they had to have found something: many patients with substantial pain. Pain that necessitated treatment, a need that was perhaps as equally contributed to by doctors' existing maxims to ease suffering as by pharmaceutical representatives who professed to have exactly what they needed to safely do so. Furthermore, this case against suffering was built in part by the fact that the treatment of *any* pain emerged from the palliative care movement, specific to the treatment of end-of-life pain. One of the major principals of palliative care, as it was led and developed by the British nurse Cicely Saunders in the 1950s and 60s, was the idea of "titrate to effect": in short, this was the idea that the correct amount of pain medication to give a patient was the amount that completely relieved pain. This distinction between the idea of pain management or treatment and the idea of pain management as only the complete eradication of pain has had enormous implications. "Titrate to effect," when practiced in a population of patients for an implicitly limited amount of time, will mean that the long-term effects of pain management as the complete cessation of pain — as provided by opioid painkillers — will never become apparent. Now, in asking whether this is about pain, desire, or suffering, one must also ask whether the relief of pain will or has truly relieved suffering, or extended it.[2]

2   Marcia L. Meldrum, "A Capsule History of Pain Management," *Journal of the American Medical Association* 290, no. 18 (2003): 2470–75, https://doi.org/10.1001/jama.290.18.2470; Cicely Saunders, "Into the Valley of the Shadow of Death: A Personal Therapeutic Journey," *British Medical Journal* 313, no. 7072 (December 1996):

Today, it is commonly stated that 100 million Americans live with chronic pain, or that "by some estimates…approximately one third of the adult population in the United States" is affected by chronic pain,[3] or that "more than 116 million Americans have pain that persists for weeks to years,"[4] or that "many tens of millions of people in the United States suffer persistent pain due to diverse problems."[5] To discuss the experiences of these people, or pain patients, we have a wide variety of words (awful, torturous, dull, throbbing, etc.) that mask the fact of what is actually an extreme deficit of narratives into which these words can fit. We have really only one narrative with which to talk about pain: the one in which pain is good when what doesn't kill you makes you stronger, even when the actual lived experience of it can only ever be expressed as "the worst" (a huge loss, unending torture, agony) and the best, most meaningful, and acceptable pain is the one that is over. The ultimate narrative of pain is the overcoming of it told in retrospect. This is the pain and conception of it that I mean when, throughout, I have been saying that the opioid epidemic is about what is and is not being called pain. What is not currently being called pain is addiction; a pain that generates a desire to seek out and take opioids; pain that is part of a chronic, messy, rare, or otherwise difficult (to describe, to commonly know) illness; pain that is generated or shaped by factors, socioeconomic, emotional, or political, generally seen only as "external" (and which may include things like access to food, medical care, transportation, and so on); any pain that

1599–1601, http://hdl.handle.net/10822/898833.

3   Perry G. Fine, "Long-Term Consequences of Chronic Pain: Mounting Evidence for Pain as a Neurological Disease and Parallels with Other Chronic Disease States," *Pain Medicine* 12, no. 7 (July 2011): 996–1004, at 996, https://doi.org/10.1111/j.1526-4637.2011.01187.x.

4   Philip A. Pizzo and Noreen M. Clark, "Alleviating Suffering 101 — Pain Relief in the United States," *New England Journal of Medicine* 366, no. 3 (January 2012): 197–99, https://doi.org/10.1056/NEJMp1109084.

5   Bruce Goldman, "Study Reveals Brain Mechanism Behind Chronic Pain's Sapping of Motivation," *Stanford University Medicine News Center,* July 31, 2014, https://med.stanford.edu/news/all-news/2014/07/study-reveals-brain-mechanism-behind-chronic-pains-sapping-of-mo.html.

does not end and cannot be expected to. It would therefore be perhaps more accurate to discuss, here, not "pain" (within this exclusionary yet prototypical conception of it) but *the pain of pain.* By *the pain of pain* I mean to include—always—exactly the socioeconomic, political, and emotional grounding and structure of pain as such; I mean, simultaneously, the physical and biological conditions that generate the pain I feel and the circumstances of it, from the fact that it is not likely to end to the fact that I have physical and financial access to a pharmacy and pain relieving medications, that add to or detract from the physical sensation—as well as the previously noted fact that part of this financial access has, at times, been made possible by Harvard University, tied as it is through Arthur Sackler to its own substantial and situated pains. Pain, the pain of pain, contains all of this. To refer to all of this throughout the rest of the chapter, I will simply say "pain," and I will continue to ask not only about what is and is not being called pain but whether this is about pain or suffering. And whether, for instance, "pain patients," when we can see that as a deeply ableist concept (predicated as it is on an image of a healthy person, an able body, with pain somehow always kept separate from illness), is adequately containing all that pain does, or whether we need a different term, or simply a different understanding of this one.

Substance

Pain, containing so much, is quite substantial. Pain is, in fact, a substance like any other. This is not really an abstract or overly theoretical statement to make, nor is it ultimately only a metaphor (as the biology of underlying pain will demonstrate). We already talk about pain as if it were any other object, with sensible qualities (sharp, hard), that is capable of producing effects on or within us (whether emotional or physical) when we find ourselves in a material proximity to it. And this material proximity to pain, like any material proximity over time, produces biological and social effects. A material proximity to pain causes long-term neurological, emotional, social, and economic changes. Attending to each of these facets of a material proximity to pain is deeply important for the information it can add to an understanding of "pain patient." Because if, as we saw, the physical, political, socioeconomic, and biological aspects of opioids that influence patterns of addiction and substance abuse seriously complicate existing notions about the nature of addiction, freedom, desire, and pain, then the same complications will arise in relation to pain. Just as we have seen the ways that *substance abuse* is as much about the sociopolitical context of what is and is not considered abusive as it is about a neurobiological condition, the conditions of a material proximity to pain will demonstrate that pain is also, in its own ways, about what is and is not abusive, and what one can and cannot stand.

The most basic element in the substance of pain is nerves. Beyond the broader, societal categorization of pain, pain is organized clinically into four main types: nociceptive, inflammatory, dysfunctional, and neuropathic. Regardless of the type, pain is essentially an object constituted by a relationship and proximity between nerve cells and a mechanical, chemical, or thermal object. Whether between a wall and the nerves in your toe, or ulcer-causing *H. pylori* bacteria and the nerves in your stomach lining, pain is always relational. Even when the distance between two things seems incapable of generating as physical and sensible a state as pain: neuropathic pain is generally defined by the very absence of an ongoing, tissue-damaging presence, but is also often caused by what was once present, like phantom limb pain following an amputation or post-surgical pain that lasts. The relationships of pain are thus broad, long-lasting, and do not require the visible, quantifiable, or physical presence of a damaging substance or object in order to be generated; pain is therefore, like addiction, also a condition of time, of what once was and what therefore will continue to be. Particularly within neuropathic kinds of pain, the ongoing and repetitive stimulation of nerves — not unlike the ongoing and repetitive cycles of dopamine and neurotransmitter disruptions within addiction — will itself begin to perpetuate pain. This kind of reorganization of the central nervous system and the functioning of nerves is a defining feature of chronic pain, though it is also worth recognizing that neuropathic pain is not a homologous category and can include mixed types of pain, wherein central nervous system reorganization is seen concurrently with ongoing inflammation or the mechanical, bone-on-bone grinding of arthritis, for example. Pain is multiple.

Given the intrinsic necessity of nerves in facilitating a material proximity to pain, and especially given the reorganization of the nervous system seen in chronic and ongoing pain, it should not be surprising that a long-term proximity to pain produces broader neurological changes. Just as opioid addiction changes the levels of dopamine and other neurotransmitters and appears as increased and decreased activity within certain brain areas, pain also causes changes within the brain that can be measured both physically and as changes to neural activity levels. Initially, pain appears to be an increase in grey matter (the physical tissue of the brain) concurrent with increased activity in particular brain regions, generally understood to be the brain working to process an increase in incoming information from the body and nervous system.[6] Over time, however, this increase reverses itself and pain eventually produces a loss of grey matter that is equivalent to aging. Specifically, this change can be measured as a rate of 1.3 cubic centimeters of grey matter lost for every year of chronic pain. In some cases, this loss is equivalent to 10 to 20 years of normal aging.[7] Interestingly, patients with different conditions will display differences in the areas of the brain affected, although the loss of grey matter is generally seen in the dorsolateral prefrontal cortex, the anterior cingulate cortex, the amygdala, and the brainstem — or, as one study put it, the "thinking parts" of the brain. More kindly, this pattern of brain changes can be described as "progressive alterations in brain connections, molecular biology, chemistry, and structure, with behavioral consequences… [due to changes in areas] involved in… cognition, motor planning and working memory."[8] These alterations have also been found

6   For a general overview of the physiology of chronic pain, see Judy Foreman, *A Nation in Pain: Healing Our Biggest Health Problem* (Oxford: Oxford University Press, 2014).

7   Northwestern University News, "Chronic Pain Shrinks 'Thinking Parts' Of Brain," November 23, 2004, https://www.northwestern.edu/newscenter/stories/2004/11/chronic.html.

8   David Borsook, "A Future Without Chronic Pain: Neuroscience and Clinical Research," *Cerebrum: The Dana Forum on Brain Science*

to be influenced by or concurrent with augmented functioning of brain areas (distinct from grey matter loss) directly related to psychomotor capabilities, memory, and executive functioning, such as the finding that "interruptions in memory traces" may play a role in producing some of the cognitive disruptions associated with chronic pain, like changes to attention or short-term memory.[9] Other research has found neural mechanisms, specifically pertaining to the level and functioning of neurotransmitters, that may account for specific emotional effects of chronic pain. One such study found that neural changes associated with chronic pain in the nucleus accumbens, a deep-brain structure, affected the working of the neurotransmitter galanin; together, given that the nucleus accumbens plays a major role in modulating reward-seeking behavior, this suggests that there is a neurological basis for the lack of motivation patients with chronic pain frequently report.[10]

When controlling for factors such as age and gender, it has also been found that pain duration, even more than pain intensity, has the strongest effect on cognitive functioning. Or, what is ill in chronic illness is time. While concurrent aspects of chronic pain like sleep disturbances or opioid use may also contribute to the observed cognitive changes, there is mounting evidence to suggest that chronic pain should be considered a neurodegenerative disorder. The policy and treatment implications of such a sentiment are not dissimilar from those proposed by the statement that addiction, too, is a chronic relapsing and remitting brain disease. Because it means that disease-specific treatment — or substance-specific, abstinence-specific treatment — will not be enough, but should instead be complemented by treatment that responds directly to the neurological conditions of a person with chronic pain. While many recent findings about the neurology of chronic pain may point to different paths for research in neuro-specific medical treatments, there is also evidence to suggest that treatment need not be invasive, intensive, or drug-driven: studies have also found that practices including yoga and mindfulness

(2012): 7, http://www.ncbi.nlm.nih.gov/pmc/articles/PMC3574803/.
9 Fine, "Long-Term Consequences of Chronic Pain," 997–98.
10 Goldman, "Study Reveals Brain Mechanism."

can reverse some of the changes in grey matter associated with chronic pain. And how similar, in a way, this is to medical maintenance treatment of opioid addiction. Because in the absence of an ability to directly and completely remove the harmful substance at hand, whether opioids or pain, it is still possible to intervene within the physical substrate that substance is situated within, wherein the physicality of yoga can replace, augment, the physicality of pain and the materiality of methadone can exist simultaneously, positively, with the neural materiality of an opioid addiction. Pain is multiple.

Nor is pain, even chronic pain, necessarily permanent. Unlike aging, it has been found that in at least some patients these neural changes can be partly reversed. A study of people with osteoarthritis of the hip, a condition in which pain can be completely gone following a total hip replacement, found subsequent increases in the grey matter of affected areas of the brain following such a surgery.[11] This should not, however, be reason to simply continue considering neural plasticity to be an unceasingly positive attribute, a commonly expressed view. While certainly remarkable, plasticity is neither positive nor negative and could instead be seen in conjunction with the discussed concept of allostatic load, a change that neural plasticity contributes to. Or, whether described as "equivalent to aging," a loss of the "thinking parts" of the brain, a sterile clinical matter of an increase or decrease in grey matter volume, or a change in the allostatic load and capacity to bear of a person in pain, the neurological effects of a proximity to pain are also always a way to describe what one can and cannot stand, what one may not even be aware of needing to stand, and what one may not need to stand forever.

Of course, in no way are neurological changes like those detailed above happening within some sort of isolated brain or person, in an emotional and social vacuum — despite the fact that many neurological studies read as if this were exactly the

11 Rea Rodriguez-Raecke, Andreas Niemeier, Kristin Ihle, Wolfgang Reuther, and Arne May, "Brain Gray Matter in Chronic Pain is the Consequence and Not the Cause of Pain," *Journal of Neuroscience* 29, no. 44 (November 2009): 13746–50, https://doi.org/10.1523/JNEUROSCI.3687-09.2009.

situation. Just as nerves are set into the scaffolding of the nervous system, pain is a substance in a larger matrix. "Chronic pain has been associated with increased rates of major depressive disorder, suicidal ideation, and suicide attempts."[12] Patients with chronic pain frequently report sleep disturbances, anxiety, and depression. Patients with chronic pain report suffering.

However, I am less interested in adding to what is already an extensive body of literature concerning the nature of suffering and pain and more so in attending to the deeply pragmatic yet less frequently noted material and economic residues of pain. Before moving fully into a consideration of these residues, I feel it is important to account for the structure of this discussion as such. Because in refusing to attend to suffering — or, really, to attend only to pain-as-suffering — what I am also saying is: what's so bad about pain? If pain is an object like any other, and particularly within this context of pain patients and chronic illness-related pain, when we are discussing pain that is not war, torture, or otherwise violence at the hands of another, is there not an ethical imperative to attend to the ways that pain, *this pain* — my pain — is not the worst? This is not to say that physical pain and the pain of an illness, accident, or injury is not painful or that the physical experience of having been tortured is worse than the physical experience of having had an awful car accident (if one truly wanted to venture a comparison of the two). Rather, asking *what's so bad about pain?* is an important rhetorical, theoretical, and ethical move in that it relinquishes ties to multiple damaging narrative constructions of pain.

First and foremost, *what's so bad about pain?* is an insertion into and also the driving apart of the dichotomy between pain patients and addicts. Throughout the opioid epidemic, its media coverage, its governmental and medical responses, and our ongoing understanding of these situations, this dichotomy has reigned rhetorically supreme. From prescribing guidelines and prescription monitoring programs to the distribution of medical maintenance treatment and research into new forms of pain management, we have seen the ways that consistent prioritization of the pain of pain patients has directly contributed to the social,

12 Fine, "Long-Term Consequences of Chronic Pain," 996.

medical, and legal denigration of those with opioid addictions, as well as those patients with harder-to-treat, messier, incorrect types of illness-related pain. Because pain that is accidental, genetic, cancer-related, or otherwise seen as *natural* is consistently privileged — and rhetorically and culturally reinforced as *the worst* — and thus as deserving not only of the mild-sounding "management" but of complete eradication via a drug that is exactly its name, a *painkiller,* there was little opposition to the practice of widespread opioid prescribing for all kinds of physical pain in the 1990s and early 2000s. Because pain that is seen as self-inflicted, morally reprehensible, avoidable, and otherwise *unnatural,* the pain of addiction, is consistently the object of law enforcement and social regulation instead of medical treatment and social support, existing evidence-based medical treatment for addiction is withheld from those who would benefit from it via geographic and socioeconomic regulatory systems that make treatment centers sporadic and inaccessible. It is this dichotomy and the hierarchy of pain it operates (within, in the name of, and as) that reinforces the medico-legal distinctions between pain patients as people with *true* pain (deserving of free access to relief) and criminals who engage in behaviors like doctor shopping and pharmaceutical diversion only under the sign of pain. Prescribing guidelines, if necessarily based on other demographic attributes like age or weight, should not include further guidelines within them for determining whose pain matters more. If we can clearly see the consequences of this kind of thinking when it comes, for instance, to identifying the racial disparities of pain treatment (predicated as those ideas are or have been on the belief that the pain of people of color is less than, less genuine, than that of white people), then why should disparities based on other demographic attributes — like the etiology of pain — persist? It is these rhetorics of true/false and natural/unnatural pain that only criminalize certain behaviors while failing to recognize the equally present pain that underlies them.

"Pain patients" is thus a concept removed not only from the reality of illness and disability, because of its reliance on and perpetuation of the image of an able body with pain, but removed as well from the physical reality and experience of actual people with pain. As a rhetorical device set within a structure predicated on a hierarchy of suffering, of creating and reinforcing systemic institutions based on concepts of whose pain matters, "pain patients" is no more representative of the lived experiences of individuals than any other symbolic and rhetorical icon is. As the supremacy of this suffering — that it is definitional, subject-forming, and subject-affirming; that it creates, in short, pain patients as it simultaneously affirms their right to relief — is continually reasserted through mass media, medical, and governmental narratives; it becomes embedded within and perpetuates ultimately unequal social relations predicated upon it. This is not about medical treatment alone, nor is it about media narratives. This is about citizenship. We have seen the ways in which attitudes about addiction and, in particular, its relationship to material objects and temporal constructs have augmented the forms of citizenship that are available to addicts within the opioid epidemic. In other words, we have seen the ways that a material proximity changes the nature of and access to freedom; it should therefore not come as a surprise to see that a material proximity to pain likewise contributes to the construction of citizenship available to the person in pain. A pain patient is only able to maintain their full citizenship because the sociopolitical and medical construction of this idea makes the right to relief central to the figure of the pain patient and implicitly dependent on the maintenance of and return to an able body; it is ultimately only the able-bodied person who has access to full citizenship. Yet when these rights and this relief are equally constituted by forms of biocapital from pharmaceutical advertising to submission within prescription monitoring programs, and when the focus on complete relief necessitates the diversion of resources that could be used to investigate and apply aforementioned non-invasive, non-drug-driven practices of pain management that may be safer and more beneficial than existing widespread opioid use — do these rights actually produce freedom? Or are they, ultimately, by functioning "as access; as markers of power...as organization of social space," a way of further extending and cementing the hierarchy of pain such rights are predicated on?[13]

13 Wendy Brown, *States of Injury: Power and Freedom in Late Modernity* (Princeton, NJ: Princeton University Press, 1995), 97.

Asking *what's so bad about pain?* is thus a complete refusal to
continually assert (what is taken as) the fact that pain is always
and only suffering which is always and only subject-forming
and subject-affirming. Because, without making this refusal
clear, we remain stuck in a realm in which the physical, organic,
accidental, genetic, or otherwise assumed "natural" pain of the
pain patient remains on a higher moral plane than the pain of a
person abusing and addicted to opioids — while continuing to
neglect the lived experiences of people with pain who, by being
unable to maintain or ever return to an able body, are implicitly
excluded. Yet the substance, the opioids, circulating between the
groups is identical: I wish to remain instead in a realm of the
identical and the horizontal wherein moral (and concurrent legal
and medical) ideas are not predicated on a hierarchy of whose
pain matters more. Saying *what's so bad about pain* does exactly
this. While it may seem to imply an attitude in which people
with pain should simply "get over it," that no illness or injury
related pain is really *that bad,* this sentiment actually counter-
acts damaging historical ideas about the subject-forming and
subject-affirming nature of pain, as encapsulated in the early
20th-century idea that the "higher the life, the keener is the sense
of pain."[14] Conceptualizing pain as an object — an object like
any other, like any other substance, like opioids — situates it as
something that can be encountered and present within anyone's
life. Situating pain in this way, horizontally instead of vertically,
it cannot simultaneously be said that some people are more or
less able to encounter, to know, to feel pain than others. And
this horizontality further limits the applicability of other damaging narratives, like the deeply rooted idea that people in pain
are unable to accurately communicate their own experiences and
sensations: this is the frequently noted "world unmaking" quality of pain, as epitomized by Elaine Scarry's landmark study *The
Body in Pain.*[15] However: do you have to own exactly the same

14 Joanna Bourke, "This Won't Hurt a Bit: The Cultural History of
    Pain," *New Statesmen,* June 19, 2014, 15–19, at 15, https://www.
    newstatesman.com/culture/2014/06/wont-hurt-bit-cultural-history-
    pain.
15 Elaine Scarry, *The Body in Pain: The Making and Unmaking of the*

chair or book or table, or have gone to the exact same beach or forest or library as I have, to understand what these objects and encounters are? *What's so bad about pain?* is a refusal to work from a position predicated on an inability to communicate and understand one another's pain. This is, after all, an epidemic. No one has the luxury of thinking themselves un-involved, unable to understand or otherwise unable to participate emotionally and empathetically. Pain is not world "unmaking." It is always already world-making, it is our world, because it is a fact of life.

Furthermore, not only does *what's so bad about pain?* relinquish a belief in the supremacy of suffering as such (as such, that is, within existing cultural and social notions of it) but it relinquishes a belief in the supremacy of *my* suffering. By refusing to continually reassert the supremacy of my own suffering, I am also refusing to continually reassert the supremacy of an individual and the pain of an individual. Destabilizing the scene of a singularly-constructed, whole, able, capable individual can destabilize the intense scene of biocapitalization that surrounds it. Without such a reliance on the supremacy of the individual within conceptions of pain, we could instead, and in addition, attend to the systemic nature of pain and its socioeconomic pressures. Or, if one did not need to conceive of a pain patient as an inherently able-bodied individual (or one that can and should maintain hope of a complete return to an able body), then more attention, resources, and research could be paid to the pain management applications of practices focused on decreasing instead of eradicating pain, though they may risk lower profits.

I do not mean to sound ungenerous when trying to make this point strongly. Again, I am not saying that pain is not painful, or that people with pain should simply get over it. Rather, I am saying that pain *is* that bad when constructed narrowly within these ideals of individuality and able-bodied-ness. What is more difficult than managing pain is managing relations to the notion of what it is to be able and what it is to continuously (have to) strive to not be in pain. What is more difficult than managing pain is managing relations to the fact that it will not end. I say *what's so bad about pain* because it is not pain itself, not my pain,

World (Oxford: Oxford University Press, 1985).

but the fact that it produces the feeling of unfreedom. What makes all of this work more difficult, what comes to constitute unfreedom and states of citizenship predicated upon normative concepts of disability, is the continued assertion that the only goal of medicine, and therefore of the individuals who practice it and are served by it, and therefore of sick people, should be the return to and maintenance of an able body. But particularly given the long-term neurological and biological effects of chronic pain, that simply is not attainable. It is far more attainable (and, I would argue, realistic) to work instead towards a better understanding of the systemic pressures that shape many people's experiences of pain, that indicate the ways that pain is deeply multiple and rhizomatic, and that recognize that the physical inabilities produced by or tied to pain are simply an instance of what it means to live in relation to an object. It is a difficult object, nonetheless, to discuss as much as to live with: consider the following, from Dr. Atul Gawande's book *Being Mortal: Medicine and What Matters in the End,* an intensive look at end-of-life care:

> For many, such talk, however carefully framed, raises the specter of a society readying itself to sacrifice its sick and aged. But what if the sick and aged are *already* being sacrificed — victims of our refusal to accept the inexorability of our life cycle?[16]

The comparison to processes of aging within discussions of pain here and in neuroscience are telling: we need to stop considering pain and chronic pain to be *like* normal processes, and recognize that they simply are *the* normal processes. The way to move from the centrality of the able body in conceptions of individuality, suffering, and constructs of pain patients is not to replace it with the centrality of the disabled body — to reassert, that is, the supremacy of suffering — but to dissolve the concept of ability itself. Pain is normal.

This work, the work of saying *what's so bad about pain?,* is a fundamental step in the project of what it means to *live with* because it necessarily recognizes that pain, as an object like any

16 Atul Gawande, *Being Mortal: Medicine and What Matters in the End* (New York: Metropolitan Books, 2014), 20.

other, is something that one can be *with* as in any other material proximity. The importance of this — both for living with pain and for living with other substances, like opioids — lies in the way that "with" recognizes multiplicity (and the presence of two or more physical things) while it also recognizes and constructs instrumentality, because, at a basic level, "with" is a metaphor. "With" is the metaphor of sentences like: "I'm going out for a drive with Sally," when Sally is the name of a car. "With" is the conduit through which objects become companions.[17] Even just through the nature of instrumentality, "with" becomes the perfect metaphor of what it is to have chronic pain and illness. Because instrumentality suggests definition, suggests concreteness — and concrete is always a mixture.

In some ways, if only to make clearer the deep connection between what it is or what it can be like to live with substances as much as with pain, *what's so bad about pain?* could also be read as akin to the statement and sentiment that begins any process of Alcoholics or Narcotics Anonymous: a recognizing of and giving up to a higher power. Although *living with* is (could be) more of a giving of, giving together, or not giving in.

Not giving in, that is, to the higher regulatory powers of bio-capital, as discussed, that simultaneously value pain even as these forms of power denigrate it. Because the only truly valuable form of pain within a complex capitalist construction predicated on the circulation of power, substances, economic and social validity via systemic institutions that must cloak this circulation even as it is perpetuated, that must perpetuate it under the name of higher moral order (whether via "the children," "the economy," "the family," or similar tropes), is the rhetorical power of the body in pain. The body in pain is used as an image, an icon, and a trope to sway, to cloak, and to construct the very institutions that perpetuate pain. While it may be said that these systemic forms are in a complex and new formation within our late capitalist moment, it is also true that this rhetorical power has, in one way or another, always existed and always been used for political gains. During the French Revolution, for instance, it was "the

17 George Lakoff and Mark Johnson, *Metaphors We Live By* (Chicago: University of Chicago Press, 1980).

moral directives of [Romantic] sensibility...[which drove a form of] highly politicized, highly effective, and highly dangerous mode of argument, one that could win one's case rhetorically by transferring the moral weight of the pained body to the side one wants it to be on."[18] This form of argument was utilized equally by pro- and anti-Revolutionary forces. Ultimately, this is the goal of saying *what's so bad about pain?*, in that it is a refusal to recognize this rhetorical force and a refusal to utilize it here. Even or especially because doing so means refusing to prioritize my own pain within the context of an epidemic of both pain and abuse that is killing thousands. So, while I can still say that "I am a pain patient," and I can say that "I have pain everyday," that this pain is bad, or that "many thousands of people are living with pain," and "many thousands of people are dying of opioid overdoses," it is also true that the only truly accurate and responsible thing I can say is: I take opioids. I have pain. "The pursuit of political freedom...[requires] sustained willingness to risk identity, both collective and individual."[19]

The Industry of Pain

These processes of biocapitalization that produce the construct "pain patient" are particularly blatant within the material and economic residues of pain. As the neurological, emotional, and social effects of chronic pain result in situations such as an inability to leave one's house, difficulty traveling, and other physical obstacles, it should not be surprising that many of the effects of pain are economic; if you have difficulty leaving your house, or standing for long periods of time, how much of what kind of job can you realistically hold? And who hires the worker who cannot work? Whether expressed through metrics concerning lost labor, lost wages, or lost income, economic disparities between sick and non-sick people exist for every age group.[20] Pain, like many

18 Steven Bruhm, *Gothic Bodies: The Politics of Pain in Romantic Fiction* (Philadelphia: University of Pennsylvania Press, 1994), 23.

19 Brown, *States of Injury*, 25.

20 Lewis Kraus, "2016 Disability Statistics Annual Report" (Durham, NH: University of New Hampshire, 2017), 19, figure 22, https://

substances, is, more broadly, money itself. "The total financial costs of this epidemic [of pain] are $560 billion to $635 billion per year... The annual U.S. expenditures related to pain (including direct medical costs and lost wages) are higher than those for cancer, heart disease and diabetes combined."[21] And here, between "direct medical costs" and "lost wages," we can see how pain moves seamlessly between expense (to those that have it) and profit (to those that treat it, manufacture objects used in the treatment of it, or manage the companies who manage the treatment of it). Pain is money in the form of pharmaceuticals, medical technology and development budgets, healthcare spending (both private and public), the quantity of mass media attention (and therefore concurrently advertising budgets) paid to stories involving pain, and the twin industries of alternative healthcare objects and the industry related to substances, particularly food, that are in one way or another preventative. Pain, in short, is a multibillion-dollar industry — an industry of pain, apparent pain, and fear of pain. And how far and broadly this industry extends, which could include anything from the entire industry now devoted to gluten-free foods, for instance (and the fear of gastrointestinal pain or embarrassment) to the nearly imperceptible objects necessary for the objects of the pain industry: who manufactures the plastic bottles of pharmaceuticals? Where does this money begin and end?

And how much I think about this money when I think about what it means to say *an epidemic of pain* or *an epidemic of chronic pain.* Particularly given its being situated within the context of the opioid epidemic, there are striking similarities between the fears expressed about and through an epidemic of pain to historic fears expressed about and through perceived epidemics of drug use. In pre-WWI-era Britain, for instance, drug use was reframed as a war issue precisely because of the relationship between drug use and labor as constituted by fear: industrialized and mechanized warfare needs the support of a labor force made up of bodies that are themselves easily mechanized

disabilitycompendium.org/sites/default/files/user-uploads/2016_AnnualReport.pdf.

21 Pizzo and Clark, "Alleviating Suffering 101," 197.

and dependable. "A drunken field hand is one thing, a drunken railroad brakeman quite another."[22] Thus I cannot help thinking *an epidemic of lost labor* when I hear "an epidemic of pain;" I cannot help but hear that it is not pain — as in, the experience of it, the pain of pain — that matters but the money my pain costs others. The opioid epidemic is its costs.

This history of these costs is the history of pain management. The anger and rage I feel, that is more or less clearly expressed when discussing rhetorics, the body in pain, lost labor, and socio-economic practices, is also tied to the history of pain management. Because, especially as pain can be an object like any other, pain is not the problem. Pain is a thing that happens. Even on a basic level, rhetorical and legal constructions of rights based on ability are not the entire problem. The problem underlying so many of these other assumptions, practices, and systems lies in pain management itself and the beliefs that motivate that practice. Saying that pain is a thing that happens may, now, sound harsh, ungenerous, and otherwise remarkable but the fact is that, historically, pain *was* just a thing that happened. Pain was a thing that happened to many people, to so many that it was expected and ordinary and not automatically the object of intensive medical care with the aim of complete eradication. The fact that pain is no longer a prominent, expected, and normal part of life for the majority of people is due not only to obvious positive achievements in medicine that have reduced the incidence of illness and injury, but the fact that these achievements also laid the groundwork for a culture in which the only normal state is the body with no pain, no other illness. And yet: is it human biology that has significantly changed over the past hundred years, or culture? One could argue that it is, actually, human biology, given that what we consider to be old age (with many people now living well into their seventies and eighties) is a new phenomenon. This is true, but it is more accurate to point out that it has not been life *span* that's changed but life *expectancy*. In the late 19th century, for instance, average life span was about 76 years old, comparable to today; the life expectancy, however,

22 David Courtwright, *Forces of Habit: Drugs and the Making of the Modern World* (Cambridge, MA: Harvard University Press, 2001), 178.

was much lower. Similarly, we will find within the history of pain management that what has changed more dramatically than pain itself is our expectations.

History

The history of pain is the history of relief. Opium has been the predominant form of pain relief for centuries: in the form of laudanum after 1680, as mass-manufactured morphine after 1820, as intravenous morphine after 1855, as newer synthetic opioids after both World Wars, as abuse-deterrent formulations after 2000. This time span has, of course, seen the development of other forms of medical treatment of pain, with a notable focus on treatment of acute pain. In 1848, ether gas was introduced as an anesthetic to be used during surgeries, childbirth, and dental work, though physicians had differing ideas about how much should be administered to any given patient. During this time period, utilitarian ideas about the aim of reducing the greatest amount of pain within a society circulated amid existing Romantic ideals about the nature of pain, suffering, and the supremacy of individual experiences, and contributed to "an extended debate over the ethics of operating on an unconscious patient…[because of] the possibility that relief from pain might actually retard the healing process."[23] Despite any such qualms, new forms of pain relief continued to be sought and when, in 1917, the painkiller aspirin (first released in 1899) became a generic and freely available, over-the-counter drug, it quickly became the drug of choice, over opiates, for mild pain. Given that 1917 also saw the passage of the Harrison Narcotic Act, which seriously restricted the distribution of certain substances, like morphine, ensuring that they would be much less readily available, the availability of aspirin was well-timed. Even before this act was passed, fears about the overuse of opiates and the dangers of iatrogenic addiction (addiction among patients prescribed opiates for pain) persisted; the opioid epidemic is what has already happened. It was these fears, in part, which led to the 1929 formation of the Committee on Drug Addiction, subsequently under the aegis of

23 Meldrum, "A Capsule History of Pain Management," 2470.

the National Institute of Health. The Committee's aim was to develop and test new drugs in the hopes of finding a substance as strong as an opiate but without any damaging side effects. For chronic pain, treatment options in the mid-20th century were both more limited and more drastic. Nerve blocks were a procedure of choice and could be performed either through a series of injections of an anesthetic (like procaine, the precursor to cocaine) or through surgeries involving the crushing or resection of nerves; these procedures were often severely disabling.

While World War II saw the development of many new synthetic painkillers, it was also a period of equally important developments in the conceptualization of pain, from the observations of Henry K. Beecher on the differences between reports of pain by soldiers on the battlefield as opposed to those of his patients at Massachusetts General Hospital (subsequently becoming an initial understanding of the placebo effect) to the experiences of John Bonica, whose time as an anesthesiologist at Madigan Army Hospital inspired his pursuit of a multi-disciplinary model of pain management. This latter development, in particular, mirrored the almost concurrent development of palliative care that was taking place in Great Britain, to which we will return. After mentioning one final development, that of the proposal of the gate control theory of pain by Ronald Melzack and Patrick Wall in 1965, I could end a history of pain management in the mid- to late-20th century and not be remiss in doing so. While there have been any number of developments in the understanding of the physiology and neurology of pain, as discussed above, there have not, particularly, been new developments in the management of physical pain. The 1982 World Health Organization ladder of pain treatment options remains, albeit with revisions, the primary model of pain management today.

Any history of pain management, however brief, is incomplete without an understanding of the closely related fields of end-of-life care and palliative care. Though similarities and influences among the three fields often go unremarked, they have always been present. Beginning with end-of-life care, one can see why it may be that this field is not often linked to pain management: it is a relatively new practice. The term given to medical care practiced during the period of old age and related infirmity that many experience, end-of-life care has only been developed as old age itself has developed. As noted, life expectancy has increased dramatically over the past 100 years and with it has come a set of experiences that we are still, relatively, unsure how to handle — particularly given what a reversal this represents from even very recent patterns of death. "As recently as 1945, most deaths occurred in the home. By the 1980s, just 17 percent did."[24] Instead of dying of sudden causes (e.g., a heart attack or stroke), many people die only at the end of protracted illnesses or a series of old age-related conditions which send them to the hospital. Where this shift becomes most complicated is in the medical and cultural response to it, which have been deeply shaped by the belief that any and all conditions — even those most normal and expected conditions of old age — should be the object of medical interventions. Pragmatically, this belief results in instances like the data which shows that 25 percent of all Medicare spending is allotted for the 5 percent of patients who are in their final year of life.[25] While one may argue that the increased attention to the dying (and therefore, presumably, to their suffering) is a positive change, the consequences of increased medical intervention are not straightforward. For instance, elderly patients who receive more than four different prescription drugs, likely for conditions from arthritis and blood pressure to vision loss and Alzheimer's, are more likely to experience falls than patients with fewer medications. A fall, for an elderly person who may already be experiencing multiple other conditions, can be catastrophic. Even the hospitalization possibly following a fall — again, presumably only a positive thing — can itself become, through hospital-acquired infections, pneumonias, or bedsores, a scene of debility and death. To counteract such a sequence of common events, some within the medical profession point to the importance and success of geriatricians, who are trained to care for the conditions of old age in a way that may more closely mirror the language of hospice care than that of hospitalizations: maintenance, comfort, reduction. Furthermore, patients near the end of their lives who choose hospice care outright have actually

24 Gawande, *Being Mortal,* 15.
25 Gawande, *Being Mortal,* 186.

been shown to have more positive experiences (across multiple measures like pain reduction and even length of life) than those who find themselves in intensive care; even the family members of patients who die in hospice report fewer instances of major depression six months after their loved one's deaths than those who experienced a death of a loved one in the hospital. Without in any way implying that end-of-life experiences should not be tended to and cared for, it is possible to point out the harm that can come from an approach which values and relies on medical intervention above all else. This is because what such medical practices fail to attend to is that, beyond pain relief or postponement of death, what might matter most to a patient is not the same as what might matter most to a doctor. A patient, for instance — perhaps, actually, many people — might be willing to have less time left if it meant that the time they did have could be spent at home, where they are as able as possible to participate in the activities that they have found rewarding throughout their life. And it is within these conflicting desires that so much of the harm that can be done within end-of-life care happens. The impulse towards intensive medical intervention does not take into account what may be a much more realistic image of end-of-life experiences, in that this impulse guides both doctors and their patients away from the realization that "our reverence for independence takes no account of the reality of what happens in life: sooner or later, independence will become impossible. Serious illness or infirmity will strike…. If independence is what we live for, what do we do when it can no longer be sustained?"[26] How do you *live with*?

When *living with* becomes nearly impossible, palliative care can be given. Pioneered by the British nurse Cicely Saunders in the 1950s and 60s, palliative care is the term for treatment administered to the terminally ill and dying — not only those who may die in old age. Opening the first hospice in the late 1950s, Saunders developed her treatment programs with several key concerns in mind, primarily pain relief. Her treatment of the dying was guided mainly by the concept of "titrate to effect": this is the belief that the correct amount of pain medication to give

26 Gawande, *Being Mortal*, 35.

was the amount that completely relieved the pain of the person. In Saunders's case, this medication would have been mainly that which is called the Brompton cocktail, a mixture of alcohol with either morphine or heroin, though later intravenous morphine would become the mainstay of palliative care. Her work was hugely influential and the later half of the 20th century saw a dramatic rise in the opening of hospices throughout the world.

By the late 1990s and early 2000s, palliative care and end-of-life care — in combination with aforementioned factors like pharmaceutical advertising to doctors and consumers, the development of "safe" opiates, and the adoption of pain as a fifth vital sign — have had profound implications for medical practice itself and for patients' expectations, particularly because of two key components of these practices. The first, and most pragmatic, is the way "titrate to effect" has been carried over from the practice of acute pain management in terminally ill patients into the treatment of both acute and chronic pain in any patient. The obvious implications of this when it comes to opioids is that the long-term effects of pain relief via these drugs will not be apparent in a person who is only taking opioids for an inherently limited time. This practice has only been cemented by the broader beliefs of end-of-life care, in which medical intervention — titrated to effect, as it were — is the necessary course for any and all physical experiences, even those (like aging or pain) that are, actually, completely biologically normal and expected. We struggle so much with pain because we have struggled so much with how to die. We deliberate over the relative benefits of hospitalization over hospice care, because we are so far removed from the realities of pain and illness that it is difficult to see and understand the things that may be more important than complete cessation of these experiences. We want complete relief from pain, even when pain arises in illnesses or injuries — like arthritis, for instance — that will not result in our actual deaths, because we do not believe that pain, like death, is something that we not only *can* live with, but *must* live with. The physiology of both opioid addiction and its treatment with medical maintenance can teach us a lot about what *living with* looks like, especially when what is lived with is (or seems to be) inherently uncomfortable. At a certain point, in the deep middle of an addiction, a brain and body simply cannot persist without the presence of opioids. When medical maintenance treatment provides opioids at a steady, constant, and daily rate, a brain and body can persist. People become better. Medical maintenance allows people to live the lives they want to and can live, guided by what is valuable to them, not in spite of an addiction but, I would argue, because of it: because of what the practice of daily maintenance can teach one about living with anything, and what medical maintenance can demonstrate about the positive effects of recognizing the natural (or imposed) limitations of a body and the necessity of recognizing and fulfilling the needs these limits create. In comparison, the practice of pain management, as it is currently practiced and influenced by the related practices of end-of-life and palliative care, is guided by an implicit belief among both doctors and patients that pain is not normal; that it is not an inherent aspect of having a living body; that it is not something that, having become daily, cannot be neatly removed from a life; that it therefore demands medical treatment that completely eradicates it and does not stop until this eradication is complete. We have come nearly as far as possible from the 19th-century debates about the ethics of anesthesia: who, today, would argue that it is unethical *not* to treat pain (or not treat it to complete relief)?

This impulse towards complete eradication of pain and its consequences is, in some ways, built directly into the term "palliative care" itself. Palliative is from the Latin *palliare,* meaning "to cloak." Pain management has become the practice of who and what is cloaked, remains cloaked, and from whom. Cloaking pain from the person experiencing it is one thing, but the narrative and rhetorical expansion of this cloak in which pain itself becomes sequestered away — *a thing that sick people get, a thing that old people get* — is something else. It is as if the only way to treat or "cure" pain patients is to prevent them from being thought of as sick people, to cloak from all involved the fact that pain is (representative of) tissue damage which is (representative of) death. Ultimately all that is cloaked is the absolute normality of this.

Reconciliation

Believing that there are rhetorical, social, and political dangers embedded within the practices and discourses of palliative care and pain management does not simultaneously mean believing pain relief should be limited in scope or application. It simply means that I believe our approach to the treatment of pain needs to be paradigmatically different. For instance, I do not believe that recently proposed and passed legislation that limits opioid prescriptions for those already receiving them (that imposes upon patients regulations like extra doctor visits or prescription monitoring) will be successful in combatting either pain itself or opioid abuse. In terms of the latter, while it remains true that prescription pills are present in the majority of overdose deaths, it is also true that the far more immediate and future threat lies in the increasing availability of stronger and stronger synthetic drugs like fentanyl; attention should be paid to this develop-ment, from both a law enforcement and treatment or outreach perspective, rather than to prescribing practices themselves. In terms of pain treatment, it is obvious that limiting the single most available option for pain relief will not relieve anyone's pain. Furthermore, denying a person medication that helps them even when it may come with dangerous side effects is a slippery slope. Following this logic, there are any number of other medications and substances we could limit or ban for the same reason, from antipsychotics and sedatives to birth control and non-steroidal anti-inflammatories. Prohibition does not decrease deaths, nor is it possible to have only those "perfect" substances with no side effects in circulation, especially when it comes to substances that have concurrent positive effects, or may be the only substance readily available that attends to the material human right that is pain relief. A solution to these conflicts of pain management and pain relief — a solution, ultimately, to what is and is not being called pain and what is and is not being called desire — must be social, cultural, and conceptual fundamentally, before we can make and enact policy.

A solution must therefore become a paradigmatic shift from a focus on pain *management,* with all the implications of economics, industrial organization, and labor that "management" contains, to a focus on *living with* and a focus on *healing.* What's so bad about pain is the fact that it is expected to end. Pain management attends to these expectations and works to realize this end. But pain often does not end, and even if it does, it is likely to happen again within one's lifetime. What's so valuable about healing as a model for pain treatment is that it attends to the theoretical (broadly speaking), as much as the physical, and makes it easier to envision a field in which treatment plans are well-rounded and can include attention to community health and interpersonal relations as much as to daily practices and lifestyle changes that make pain easier to live with. Even the smallest changes can have profound implications for a person's life and, most importantly, can easily be lifelong changes. Pain treatment must be manageable *for* an individual and not only in terms of the bio-management *of* an individual, which is measured in lost labor and healthcare spending. Healing implies reduction and wholeness, not endings and eradication. This is ultimately the largest and most important project in understanding the rhizomatic structures of end-of-life care, palliative care, and pain management: the influences of the former two fields have helped create a form of pain management that is simply and only the work of managing pain. It is not the work of managing relations to pain, which takes healing and work that is as theoretical as it is physical — work that can begin to understand an *imaginative proximity* as much as a material proximity. This is one of the most important understandings we can take from end-of-life care and particularly the most recent developments in the field: the recognition of the basic importance of discussing and understanding what actually matters to a person, what their desires are for their life, and the effect that a temporal perspective has on these desires. The researcher Laura Carstensen, for example, has found profound similarities between the perspectives of ill people and elderly people, to the extent that serious illness mitigates the perspectives of youth. In a study which asked participants whether they would rather spend time with a known loved one or with someone they didn't know, who offered informative or

emotional newness, Carstensen found that young people generally chose to spend time with new people and older people chose
to spend time with loved ones. However, "among the ill, the
age differences disappeared. The preferences of a young person
with AIDS were the same as those of an old person."[27] When the
emotional, psychological, and temporal states of ill people and
elderly people are demonstrably similar, it should be intuitive
that the same things that are of value in end-of-life care — allowing people to retain as much autonomy over their lives as possible
while providing assistance with daily tasks that may have become
difficult, all the while focusing on *comfort over cure* — should also
be valued in treatment for those living with chronic illness and
pain. Valuing individual lives, desires, and experiences is what
healing looks like; it does not look like complete medical eradication of a problem. This is especially true of a problem, like pain,
that may not even be the entire or the main problem; because, in
living with, is it pain itself that is the problem or the way that pain
prevents you from engaging in certain activities? Or the way that
pain always reminds you that it may become worse? If the latter
is true, and if the pain is part of a chronic illness or otherwise
cannot be expected to end, shouldn't a solution focus not on an
improbable cessation of pain but instead on adjustments that
may make a given activity more possible? When the pain that
I experience began to effect my range of motion, I realized that
I was having near-daily anxiety about my ability to cook dinner
every night, when I am often the only person home before my
partner returns from work. While I could have chosen to start
taking more pain medication prior to cooking, I instead chose
to reorganize my kitchen and found that even moving singular
objects significantly relieved the anxiety I was having. I have not
had to increase my medication — which itself can render me suf-
ficiently drowsy to interfere with the act of cooking — because,
thanks to an hour of rearranging, I no longer have to worry about
being able to get a large pot down or pick up a heavy appliance. I
know that this will only remain true for so long, that eventually
(even if it is years from now) I will experience some other change
in pain that will create a new set of concerns or obstacles. But I

27 Gawande, *Being Mortal,* 125.

also know that inherent within this decision is a recognition that what is vital to the maintenance of my sense of autonomy is a recognition of that autonomy and independence as a *freedom with.* Choosing to make a small, manageable change that preserves my ability to engage in an activity that is important not only because it is a necessary component of daily life but, more importantly, because it allows me to continue feeling that I am providing and caring for my family, is a choice towards *living with*— towards *freedom with* — and not towards complete removal of pain. I will still be in pain while cooking, but I will at least be cooking. The recognition of the importance of autonomy as a *freedom with* should not be reserved only for the last years or months of life, because it is this recognition that provides any sense of freedom within such a situation of inherent limitations.

Is it wishful thinking to imagine that a healthcare system so predicated upon the profitability of intensive, short, and immediate procedures will be able to transform into one of holistic, socioeconomically-engaged, and individualized plans based on comfort and healing? Probably. But it is also true that on a basic level, from individual cells to complex organisms, from the way that blood clots at a wound to the actions of an immune system in the face of the flu, healing is an intrinsic function of life.

5

Opioids

I know that the periphery is the only place I can be, that I would die if I let myself be drawn into the center of the fray, but just as certainly if I let go of the crowd. This is not an easy position to stay in, it is even very difficult to hold, for these beings are in constant motion and their movements are unpredictable and follow no rhythm.... So too am I in perpetual motion; all this demands a high level of tension, but it gives a feeling of violent, almost vertiginous, happiness.

— Fanny Deleuze, quoted in *A Thousand Plateaus: Capitalism and Schizophrenia*[1]

Endogenous

We have been, up until now, at the level of the molar. We have examined the points and intersections at which opioids exist, at the largest and broadest levels: the sociopolitical systems which distribute opioids throughout the country; the economic and industrial pressures likewise contributing to this distribution;

1   Gilles Deleuze and Félix Guattari, *A Thousand Plateaus: Capitalism and Schizophrenia,* trans. Brian Massumi (London: The Athlone Press, 1988).

the legacy of stigma and biopolitics that has carried over primarily from the AIDS epidemic, which has longstanding roots in the treatment of the ill and Other; the way in which an act and experience of taking an opioid is set within this structure of the social, the political, the stigmatized; the biological and physical network operating simultaneously to construct personal and bodily experiences not only of opioid abuse or addiction but of chronic pain; the history of medicine and of law enforcement that has contributed to our current situation, creating a lack of adequate, appropriate, and accessible pain treatment options in the case of the former, and a lack of adequate, appropriate, and accessible responses to the flood of opioids throughout the United States in the case of the latter — and the systemic racism and ableism which is undeniably a part of both histories.

But what of the molecular? Although included somewhat within an understanding of the neurological conditions of a material proximity to opioids, we have not yet fully examined and recognized a fundamental state that opioids exist in, and as, at the molecular level. Because there is indeed a state in which opioids exist neither as a medication, a pill, a product, a profit, an addictive drug, a social ill, nor any other material other than exactly what they are, on the most basic level: the substance of an opioid; the substance of endorphins. Endorphins are a group of biochemicals that are naturally produced by every single human body (and many other mammals besides). As their name suggests, endorphins are morphine-like substances that arise naturally within the human body; *endorphin* names a substance of *endogenous morphine.*

The opioid epidemic is many people in the same place at the same time because it is all of us. The opioid epidemic is many people in the same place at the same time because it is centered on a substance that it is always already within all of our bodies and which, through this state of being endogenous, can deepen our understandings of what it means for conditions to be *systemic* and what it means to be within, to live within, an epidemic — one so all-encompassing, it is endogenous.

Coming to such an understanding will first necessitate a better understanding of the physiology of endorphins and the role that these substances play in our major bodily functions.

A group of chemicals secreted by the central nervous system and the pituitary gland, endorphins modulate experiences of pain by providing a form of endogenous pain relief, a relief that originates within and is produced by one's own body. A contraction of *endogenous* and *morphine,* "endorphin" refers to what is actually a group of related neuropeptides (protein-like molecules used in communication among nerve cells) whose mechanism of action can be described broadly: endorphins produce feelings of analgesia through the act of binding to opioid receptors throughout the body. These are the very same receptors involved in any experience of taking an exogenous opioid. When endorphins bind to these opioid receptors, particularly *mu*-receptors, or those which morphine binds to, they trigger a cascade of further biochemical processes involved in the transmission of pain. Which cascade is triggered will depend on where within the body the endorphin-*mu*-receptor binding takes place, and can include a tachykinin called Substance P (another kind of neuropeptide) or the neuropeptide GABA, related to the regulation of dopamine (which, as we saw in the neurophysiology of addiction, is a main component of reward circuitry within the brain); in short and in a very basic sense, endorphins feel good.

From an initial wave of analgesia following an accident to the common experience of a "runner's high," endorphins are substances fundamental to bodily experiences of pain and stress. However, their effects are perhaps felt most prominently and forcefully within the biological, social, and emotional experience commonly termed the *placebo effect* or *placebo response.*[2] The placebo response is a set of physiological mechanisms and social or personal experiences that, together, produce feelings of relief through relationships to endorphins as well as other endogenous substances, as "relief" can include both pain relief and relief from symptoms like nausea or insomnia. Despite a recent surge in research and interest, the placebo response still exists culturally

---

2   Throughout this chapter, I will be using the term *placebo response* instead of *placebo effect,* to continually highlight the interconnectedness of personal experience and biology rather than a term that, through *effect,* seems to suggest only something that happens to you and not something with which you are involved in producing.

and theoretically much as it did fifty to sixty years ago. Although the placebo has existed and been known for hundreds of years, whether under the term "mesmerism," "somnambulism," "the power of suggestion," or some similar term, the cementing of its clinical and scientific importance dates to the work of Doctor Henry Beecher. Intrigued by the differences in reports of pain between the soldiers he treated during World War II and the citizens he treated at Massachusetts General Hospital, Beecher found that, in short, context matters: the soldiers he treated reported less pain despite no less serious injuries because of the context of their experiences.[3] Among so many other less fortunate soldiers suffering far more severe injuries, a broken bone or bad burn may seem less painful. Among the lives of ordinary citizens, who are surrounded instead by normalcy and health, such injuries do appear to be the worst. Instead of initiating research into this effect — research that may have proven simultaneously its validity and its reproducibility within further clinical settings — Beecher proposed a very different application. In a landmark article, Beecher developed a model of pharmaceutical testing that has been in use ever since: the randomized control trial (RCT). Implicitly recognizing the power and threat of a placebo response — that it might be possible for a placebo response to be equal in effect to a pharmaceutical product — Beecher proposed the RCT as a way to pit drugs against placebos. In an RCT, one group of patients is given the active drug being tested, while a second group is given a placebo treatment. Given the contextual complexity of placebo responses, which can include everything from the specifics of what a doctor says to a patient down to the color of a pill, Beecher's proposal would limit the magnitude of a placebo response and better isolate and highlight the effects of the "actual" drug. Not, of course, that this is always possible: currently, "half of all drugs that fail in late-stage trials drop out of the pipeline due to their inability to beat sugar pills."[4]

3   For an overview of Beecher's work and a general explanation of various placebo responses, see Jo Marchant, *Cure: A Journey into the Science of Mind Over Body* (New York: Crown, 2016).

4   Steve Silberman, "Placebos Are Getting More Effective: Drug Makers Are Desperate to Know Why," *WIRED,* August 24, 2009, https://

As terms like "mesmerism" and "the power of suggestion" imply, there has always been a reason to simultaneously encapsulate and dismiss the way that a physical body is influenced by an imaginative, social, or otherwise seemingly "nonphysical," and therefore unreal, experience. Whether within a cultural and theoretical history influenced and structured by a Cartesian sense of mind–body separation, or a medical and cultural history predicated on the fields of psychology and psychoanalysis that regulated the effects of the mind on the body to only the hysterical and disordered, the placebo response has remained in the zone of the pseudo, the sham, the sugar pill. For Beecher, it was the implications of the placebo response within the pharmaceutical industry (and medical practice generally) that necessitated its being discredited as a real, physical mechanism and experience. This is because it was not only the fact that context mattered, that social relationships surrounding a person in pain could augment that person's perception and experience of that pain, but the implication that if this held true across contexts and was reproducible, what would remain of the role of pharmaceuticals?

The dismissal of the psychosomatic and mind–body experiences has so often come down to exactly this threat: that the recognition of the physical reality of the social, the imaginative and the emotional would discredit the pervading thought and practices of the day. In the late 18th century, mesmerism was a practice that purported to heal ill people through modulation of the magnetic and relational fluids that circulated within them, as well as through natural objects like trees; to be *mesmerized* was to be within an experience of having these "magnetic" fluids modulated by another person, a medical authority figure, even via these tertiary objects. Commissions set up by the French government at the time served to investigate and subsequently discredit the practice of mesmerism through what was the earliest use of a controlled trial, pitting the healing power of "mesmerized" trees against trees to which nothing had been done. Beyond acknowledging the fact that mesmerism and the manipulation of magnetic bodily fluids are indeed untrue, it is also important

www.wired.com/2009/08/ff-placebo-effect/.

to acknowledge that the discrediting of mesmerism was fundamental to emerging Enlightenment ideals about, in particular, the physicality of medicine: it could not be true that people could both be healed through seemingly nothing, through their minds, *and* through scientifically-proven and clinically validated techniques. One could also posit that, within the discrediting of mesmerism, the importance of validating the legality and rationality of the government (which initiated this process) over the spiritual, the faith-based, and the Church. The Church, too, participated in the regulation of mind–body experiences through its regulation of the practice of exorcisms (and its validation of only a subset of "true" exorcisms) and its subsequent regulation of experiences of miraculous or spontaneous healing at the site of Lourdes.[5]

Henry Beecher's work and move to relegate the placebo response to the psychological and emotional can be seen as firmly rooted within this history, though with an important point of departure. Beecher's work came at a time, post-WWII, of rapid pharmaceutical development and expansion with which his work was in perfect sync, and which can lead us to a more recent, 20th-century history of the relationship between mind–body experiences and, in a word, economics. In the early 20th century, New Thought referred to a school of thinking about the healing power of mind–body experiences that had grown out of the then-recent beginnings of the Christian Science movement. By the 1920s and 30s, the "power of positive thinking" narrative that emerged from this school had made its way firmly into the realms of the industrial and capitalist. Henry Ford, for instance, was a strong proponent of New Thought: "His famous comment 'If you think you can, you can. And if you think you can't, you're right,' is New Thought tailored to the no-nonsense world of young capitalist America."[6] Ford was quickly joined by sensations like Dale Carnegie, of *How to Win Friends and Influence People* fame, who adopted the power of thinking for capitalist, creative, and social gains. It should therefore not be surprising

5   Anne Harrington, *The Cure Within: A History of Mind–Body Medicine* (New York: W.W. Norton, 2008), 106.

6   Harrington, *The Cure Within,* 118.

that Beecher sought immediately to frame the placebo response in such a way as to limit its economic threat to the pharmaceutical industry and to mainstream medicine, inasmuch as he was working in a time that implicitly recognized that mind–body relationships were no longer solely medical or psychological issues, but fundamental to capitalist economics. Beyond any history of suggestion, of mesmerism, of psychoanalysis, it is perhaps this threat to pharmacological capitalism that most strongly necessitated the relegation of placebos to the unreal — and which means that this history and the placebo response at the center of it is directly related to what is and is not being called pain and what is and is not being called relief within the opioid epidemic. The idea that the relief a body itself makes possible, as produced through imaginative, social, and emotional relationships, is less real than the relief produced through a pill — a pill that, in cases like OxyContin, is worth upwards of $35 billion — is at the basis of current medical practices within the opioid epidemic. To our existing understanding of the cultural and social forces shaping what is and is not being called pain, and the relief that is and is not therefore available, we must add a sense of the economic pressures contributing similarly. This has always been the case: what is real is profitable, consumable, and reproducible; what is deemed unreal is amorphously reproducible, social, and endogenous — that is, always already outside of the realms of what can be co-opted, reproduced, and sold. The most real kind of pain is the kind that contributes to the $35 billion profit of OxyContin. The least real is the pain of a social and emotional experience of precarity that drives an increasingly close material proximity to opioids in the form of an addiction; that ultimately represents costs to the state and the community through the healthcare costs of addiction treatment, the costs of lost labor, and the costs of law enforcement. The biology and potential applications of placebo responses present an alternative to this dichotomy of real/unreal, profitable/unreal, physical/unreal. Placebo responses present a model for understanding a body and one's embodiment that operates in wholenesses instead of binaries, that creates not only physical and material proximities but always concurrently recognizes their imaginative dimensions.

Placebo Response

What, beyond fear, is it that allows us to continue believing that a placebo response is anything less than physical? Even just three initial examples provide strong evidence for the biological reality of placebo responses. Most strikingly within the context of the opioid epidemic are the many placebo studies that incorporate the use of naloxone, the opioid reversal medication: because, as even some of the earliest endorphin and placebo research demonstrated, naloxone blocks the pain relief produced in a placebo response just as it blocks the effects of an exogenous opioid. While striking, this should not be surprising, given that we know endorphins bind to the same receptors that morphine and naloxone bind to. And should there be any doubt as to the strength of these endogenous opioids, additional studies have found that "placebo-activated endogenous opioids [have] also been shown to produce a typical side effect of opioids — respiratory depression."[7] A sense of eeriness and of the uncanny that arises frequently in instances, like this, of mimicry and doubling, of repetition between what we think of as natural and what we think of as manufactured, is not uncalled for in relation to findings like this, but is perhaps unfounded: we are, after all, dealing with identical substances. Endogenous opioids, endorphins, and the opioids found in a morphine pill are not two different substances. The opioids manufactured today are derived from or based on a substance found in a plant, *P. somniferum,* that surely existed in that plant at least as long as it has existed in our bodies — and even "morphine itself has been shown to be present in [human] tissues and body fluids."[8] Placebo responses involve

---

7   Luana Colloca and Fabrizio Benedetti, "Placebos and Painkillers: Is Mind as Real as Matter?" *Nature Reviews: Neuroscience* 6, no. 7 (July 2005): 545–52, at 547; https://doi.org/10.1038/nrn1705.

8   Alistair D. Corbett, Graeme Henderson, Alexander T. McKnight, and Stewart J. Paterson, "75 Years of Opioid Research: The Exciting but Vain Quest for the Holy Grail," *British Journal of Pharmacology* 147, no. S1 (January 2006): S153–S162, at S157, https://doi.org/10.1038/sj.bjp.0706435.

substances and experiences that are as forceful and real as any involving opioids, a substance of such intense physical presence.

More recent research within the emerging field of psychoneuroimmunology further suggests the force of these endogenous substances and the placebo responses they operate within. As the term would suggest, psychoneuroimmunology is devoted to the study of the relationship between emotional and social experiences and physical functioning within a body, as mediated by "a physical connection between nerves and immune cells."[9] Placebo-related studies within this field have focused, for example, on the use of placebo treatments in relation to immunosuppressant medications. One landmark study focused on a group of patients recovering from kidney transplants. Often an exceedingly dangerous time in which the transplant recipient is at high risk for complications, including graft versus host disease, such complications are managed with immunosuppressant medications that are themselves dangerous. During the course of this study, participants were given immunosuppressants — along with a placebo treatment. Over time, the dose of the immunosuppressant was decreased while the placebo treatment was continued. The strength of immunosuppressing effect remained the same as it was at the higher dose of medication.[10] Applications such as this, in which placebos can be used to limit the use of a dangerous medication, are perhaps the most promising avenue of placebo research for patients.

But what, exactly, beyond modulation of endorphins, are the mechanisms that produce these varied effects? It is important to remember that although it is commonly referred to as placebo pain relief, there is in fact "not one single placebo effect, there are many."[11] These multiple mechanisms can be used to produce both general responses (pain relief, for instance) as well as

9 Marchant, "You Can Train Your Body into Thinking It's Had Medicine," *Mosaic,* February 9, 2016, https://mosaicscience.com/story/medicine-without-the-medicine-how-to-train-your-immune-system-placebo.
10 Marchant, "You Can Train Your Body."
11 Colloca and Benedetti, "Placebos and Painkillers."

responses that are "precise and somatotopic,"[12] occurring only in specific body parts (like a placebo analgesic hand cream). Within these placebo pills or creams, which consist of "substances that have no active ingredient," what, exactly, is producing the physiological responses found?[13]

Placebo responses are generated by expectations as those expectations are mediated by social and emotional experiences and the "terrain of medicine."[14] Or, as described by placebo researcher Fabrizio Benedetti:

> [T]he placebo is not the substance alone, but its administration together with a concomitant set of sensory and social stimuli that tell the patient that he or she is being treated…[because] humans are endowed with endogenous systems that can be activated by verbally induced positive expectations, therapeutic rituals and healing symbols and, more generally, by social expectations.[15]

Stereotypically, a placebo response is produced primarily through a doctor-patient (or nurse-patient) relationship. And, in fact, providing pain relief looks, in a doctor's brain, "a lot like the response in a patient's brain when he or she expected and perceived pain relief,"[16] but this is hardly the entire process. Those "therapeutic rituals and healing symbols" include as many different features of a placebo treatment as they do of the psychosocial context itself that can, together, be utilized to affect

12 Benedetti and Elisa Frisaldi, "Neurochemistry of Placebo Analgesia: Opioids, Cannabinoids and Cholecystokinin," in *Placebo and Pain: From Bench to Bedside*, eds. Luana Colloca, Magne Arve Flaten, and Karin Meissner, 9-14 (London: Academic Press, 2013), 11.

13 Alison Motluk, "Placebos Trigger an Opioid Hit in the Brain," *The New Scientist,* August 23, 2005, https://www.newscientist.com/article/dn7892-placebos-trigger-an-opioid-hit-in-the-brain/.

14 Ted Kaptchuk, quoted in Trisha Gura, "When Pretending is the Remedy," *Scientific American Mind* 24, no. 1 (March/April 2013): 34–9, at 36.

15 Benedetti, "Drugs and placebos: what's the difference?" *EMBO Reports* 15, no. 4 (April 2014): 329–32, at 329; https://doi.org/10.1002/embr.201338399.

16 Gura, "When Pretending is the Remedy."

the placebo response produced. It has been found that not only do some forms of placebo treatments work better for certain conditions than for others (as in the case of "pills for insomnia, shots for pain"[17]), but that everything from the color of a pill to its price can influence the response. In an example that recalls, in a striking way, some of the forces behind the rapid increase in the circulation of counterfeit opioid pills, it has been found that "placebos stamped or packaged with widely recognized trademarks are more effective than 'generic' placebos."[18] At the same time, a placebo treatment need not be necessarily complex or meticulously designed: "simply being in a US [drug] trial and receiving sham treatment now seems to relieve pain almost as effectively as many promising new drugs."[19] The sense of broadness and generality implicit in the latter example echoes other findings within placebo research, demonstrating that placebo responses can be reliably produced even when a patient *knows* that the treatment they're about to receive is a placebo. It is likely that the lack of systematic research prior to the past several decades has contributed to what often seems like a superfluity of placebo responses and influential characteristics of placebo treatment. This research could, for instance, better distinguish between what are likely to be multiple effects taking place, from the statistical phenomenon of regression to the mean to the fact that patients are likely to both enter trials at a particularly low point within their illnesses and experience spontaneous remission of symptoms.

For the case of endorphin-modulated placebo pain responses, I can offer a much more specific physiological explanation: strong expectation signals (from the rituals, "social terrain," and features of the placebo treatment itself) originate within the prefrontal cortex and send further signals to midbrain structures, which "release opioids to meet the expectation of reprieve."[20]

17 Gura, "When Pretending is the Remedy."
18 Silberman, "Placebos Are Getting More Effective."
19 Marchant, "Strong Placebo Response Thwarts Painkiller Trials," *Nature News,* October 6, 2015, https://www.nature.com/news/strong-placebo-response-thwarts-painkiller-trials-1.18511.
20 Gura, "When Pretending is the Remedy."

And it is specifically the induction of placebo pain responses through these strong expectations that help to distinguish placebos involving endogenous opioids from those involving other endogenous substances.

Placebo pain responses are the ultimate biological and social expression of *the expectation of force and the force of expectation.* Even if we acknowledge the fact that there are definite differences between the effects of pharmaceuticals and placebo treatments (seen mainly within the magnitude and variability of effect and duration), it is also true that "when a placebo is effective, the magnitude of that effect matches that of a drug."[21] Placebo pain responses are an example of what happens when what we think is about to happen — *the expectation of force* — produces physical effects — *the force of expectations* — as those expectations were shaped by social and emotional and imaginative experiences. This is not a foreign or unknowable idea and could be demonstrated even more simply by an exceedingly common experience, which is often called the "white coat effect." To explain the phenomenon in which people frequently have high blood pressure at their doctor's office (but not in other settings), the "white coat effect" proposes that anxiety is the cause of this difference. Or: a person's expectation of force as expressed through anticipatory anxiety dependent on contextual clues (from the waiting room and paperwork to the exam room and hospital gown), given the force of these expectations, produces a physical effect: high blood pressure.

Given the co-constitutive relationship between placebo responses and the expectation of force and the force of expectation, one could also describe placebo responses thusly: a placebo response operates within and is mediated by *imaginative proximities,* by an imaginative proximity to the future, constituted by one's expectations about what is about to happen. As a dimension of material proximities, and as demonstrated by the studies which show that placebos are effective whether a patient knows or doesn't know what kind of treatment they're receiving, imaginative proximities are likewise relationships within which you exist, whether you are aware of this involvement or not.

21 Benedetti, "Drugs and Placebos," 330.

Imaginative and material proximities describe physical and theoretical relations to things, and the never-ending Mobius strip of
the two.[22]

Speech Act

How can we better understand the functioning of imaginative proximities within the terrain of medicine and social and
emotional experiences? How is it that expectations are in fact
induced through interpersonal interactions, and are able to then
go on and produce physical experiences? To better understand
the function and workings of such a social terrain, we should
turn very specifically to the material bulk of what constitutes
this terrain: things that are said. That is, we will turn to a very
specific category of things that are said and things that are said
with physical and concrete effects: speech acts.

On a basic level, a speech act is a statement — an utterance — that *does* at the same time as it *says*: "the uttering of the sentence is, or is a part of, the doing of an action, which again would
not *normally* be described as, or as 'just,' saying something."[23]
The classic example is the utterance of *I do,* when said during
a marriage ceremony. When uttered within this specific context
and in response to the question "Do you take this person to be
your lawfully wedded spouse?" *I do* is an utterance that produces
the legal state of being married. Within this example are several
key details to note about speech acts. First and foremost is the
importance of context: I cannot say *I do* to my partner in our
own home, with no witnesses or legal or religious authority figures present, and expect us to actually be married. Not only is
the overall social context of a wedding important, but so is the

22 For the sake of clarity, I will use the term "imaginative proximity"
    throughout. In doing so, I do not mean to suggest that this is
    something separate from a material proximity — that is, I do not always
    consider it to be one dimension of a material proximity — but simply
    that referring to it as such will allow us to more clearly and specifically
    examine the details of this imaginative dimension.
23 J.L. Austin, *How to Do Things with Words,* 2nd edn. (Cambridge, MA:
    Harvard University Press, 1975), 6, emphasis in original.

specific presence of exactly such a legal or religious representative as a judge or priest. In order to successfully produce the state at which it aims, a speech act often depends on further utterances or actions that happen concurrently or subsequently. *I do* produces the legal state of being married when it is followed by the statement of a judge or priest that "I now pronounce you husband and wife," and is further accompanied by legal documentation like a marriage certificate and the state of not being already married. Further examples would include the naming of a ship while smashing a bottle over the side, as performed by the captain of the ship, or "I bequeath," as that utterance occurs in a will in reference to an object in the possession of the person making the statement. Again, in each case "it seems clear that to utter the sentence (in, of course, the appropriate circumstances) is not to *describe* my doing of what I should be said in so uttering to be doing or to state that I am doing it: it is to do it."[24] Speech acts are contextual and relational.

Given what we have just discussed about placebo responses, I would now add another example of a speech act or performative utterance: the placebo response and, specifically, an endorphin-modulated placebo pain response. Consider the following — even if it is hypothetical or idealized — situation of the administration of a placebo treatment: in a clinical setting, a patient is being seen by a doctor or nurse. The caregiving figure states: "I am now going to give you an injection of a pain reliever that should greatly improve your pain." Despite the subsequent injection of a biologically neutral substance, like a saline solution, the patient does indeed begin to feel pain relief. The statement "I am now going to give you an injection that will relieve your pain" is a speech act, that says as much as it does: what it does is a create a state of expectation within the patient that induces pain relief through direct and physical connections between the neurophysiology of that state of expectation and the physical substance, endorphins, that is capable of producing pain relief. Of course, like many scenarios whose successful completion depends on speech acts, this too depends on numerous other factors, including the actual action of an injection, that the doc-

24 Austin, *How to Do Things with Words,* 6.

tor and patient had even a brief but positive relationship, or that the injection was visually similar to a syringe, for instance, of morphine: exactly the factors we have already identified as being influential in producing placebo responses.

Placebo responses are a form of speech act, although certain objections to this classification may be immediately apparent. One of the first categories of infelicities that J.L. Austin himself identified — those utterances that for any number of reasons fail to completely and correctly achieve the action at hand — is the case of utterances where "one or another of its normal concomitants is *absent*. In no case do we say that the utterance was false but rather that the utterance — or rather the *act*, e.g., the promise — was void, or given in bad faith, or not implemented, or the like."[25] It could be objected that placebos are void inasmuch as they are inherently dependent on the absence of a "normal concomitant;" that is, an active drug that may normally accompany and be present in the situation of prescribing and receiving a medication or treatment in a doctor's office. But it cannot be said that nothing is being *implemented*: it is just that what is implemented remains somewhat outside the bounds of what we normally consider to be an active substance (a drug), or the substance of a promise. A deeper look at the circumstances Austin outlines for successful utterances can further clarify this response to such an objection. An utterance that successfully carries off its action will include "the uttering of certain words by certain persons in certain circumstances," in which the persons and circumstances are "appropriate for the invocation of the particular procedure invoked," and are in turn "correctly...and completely" executed by all involved, including "certain consequential conduct" such as "thoughts or feelings."[26] Furthermore, in contrast to acts which may *appear* to ascribe to these circumstances but which are ultimately unsuccessful — i.e., the utterances of actors on a stage — Austin focuses instead on acts in which the "performative utterances, felicitous or not, are to be understood as issued in ordinary circumstances."[27] It is the very

25 Austin, *How to Do Things with Words,* 10–11, emphasis in original.
26 Austin, *How to Do Things with Words,* 14–15.
27 Austin, *How to Do Things with Words,* 22.

ordinariness of the medical context surrounding the utterances of placebos and their administration that constitutes the effectiveness of a placebo response, and in a sense renders null objections along the lines of their being void or false given their predication on substances themselves seen as false: ultimately, the speech acts of a placebo response are made of this medical ordinariness and not because of the presence of any specific and *singular* object as such. Recognizing the functionality of a placebo response as first and foremost a linguistic and social act necessitates recognizing the concreteness — the biological and physical concreteness — of said act and the way that this concreteness usurps the importance of a *seemingly* more physical substance at hand, or that should be at hand — i.e., an active drug. Or, the effectiveness of an endorphin-modulated placebo pain response is initiated primarily through the social, linguistic, and emotional, and subsequently through the physical presence of a specific substance. After all, it is the presence of expectation signals within the brain induced through contextual clues that triggers the release of endogenous opioids and not the already-circulating presence of those endorphins. The expectation of force constitutes the force of expectation; the expectation of force arises through social and linguistic context.

But why should this matter, to placebos, to opioids, to the opioid epidemic? The importance and value of the idea of a speech act is twofold: first in that it provides us with an analytical and critical tool for recognizing the functionality of linguistics, the importance of what is said — and therefore what is thought and imagined — within a field that is primarily concerned with the visual, the verifiable, the resolutely physical and that in many cases, by definition, negates the physical reality of the former. Placebo responses as constituted by speech acts provide an example and model for understanding the importance of what is thought and imagined to what is biologically real and physically felt. Secondly, inasmuch as this understanding can bring us closer to an understanding of the imaginative dimensions of material proximities and the implications of these proximities not only within ourselves but within our relations to others, a placebo-speech act relationship is a tool for coming to a broader relationship between placebos, opioids, and the opioid epidemic;

especially given that the substances within placebos and within the epidemic are identical. If we can recognize linguistic statements, that an utterance like *I do* is able to produce such abstract yet definite conditions as *the legal,* we should then be able to recognize that utterances are equally capable of producing such abstract yet definite conditions as *pain relief, the biological.*

What is it that prevents us from acknowledging this recognition? What else, besides the theoretical and economic threats identified herein, prevents us from adding a sense of the biological to the sense of the legal that already exists within an understanding of speech acts? Or, if we can recognize that physical effects are indeed produced through social, emotional, and personal experiences insofar as they are mediated linguistically, then what happens to the boundaries we have long erected between "real" and "not real" pain and relief? Who pays for placebo treatments? How do insurance companies measure the effectiveness of what are essentially interpersonal relationships with biological consequences? How do we continue deciding and believing that a group of people deeply situated in relationship to opioids within an addiction is, in fact, in a relationship that is somehow less real (and therefore must be "ill" or "disordered") than the relationships of "normal" or "healthy" people — people who do not abuse their medications or are able to, seemingly, temporarily, avoid them altogether, despite the fact that biologically, endogenously, we are all already in equally real relations to the substance of opioids? With a deeper understanding and acknowledgment of the reality of placebo responses, could we really continue to operate within these same assumptions? Could we really continue to believe that the relief a body is capable of isn't real, or isn't real enough? Or, likewise, could we continue our disbelief in the idea that the emotional, social, and economic-political state of being in an addiction does not create and correspond to an equally real biological state, that the two are in fact co-constitutive and must therefore equally contribute to our understanding of "reality"? With a deeper understanding of placebo responses and speech acts, would we continue to rely solely on pharmaceutical treatments sought for complete and absolute relief of pain (yet themselves carriers of deep, endemic dangers), when such a reliance is predicated on the denial of what is so natural — pain and relief — it is always already, always endogenous, within every human body? Or would we be able to recognize that at least some unknown percentage of an experience of pain is modulated socially and emotionally as much as biologically and therefore requires treatment and support attendant to these aspects? Would we be able to fully realize that the widely circulating narratives of "once an addict, always an addict," that set up expectations for and position addiction as a permanent future, are as physically and biologically damaging as the lack of treatment options they engender?

Imaginative Proximity

And it is this latter question, in particular, that can bring us fully in relation, again, to the opioid epidemic. Because ultimately, placebo responses and speech acts are about recognizing the reality of imaginative proximities, that we exist in theoretical relationships as much as physical ones, that as biosocial relationships our material proximities always already have imaginative dimensions — and that these theoretical relationships affect not only ourselves but others. Whether I have chosen to be or not and whether I am always aware of these relationships or not, I am constantly in relation to narratives through mass media, conversations I have with friends or family, conversations I have with my doctor, people I see walking around Boston, scientific studies I read about pain management, and so forth. All of these narratives, individual statements, and even individual words shape the imaginative dimensions of my material proximity to opioids. That is, these relationships and proximities shape simultaneously what I *imagine* opioids to be; the *reality* I therefore construct around the idea and substance of opioids; and the *emotional and critical reaction* I have to these ideas. An imaginative proximity is a relationship of distance and closeness to ideas, ideals, narratives, and rhetoric that cumulatively shape the reality of a thing, a substance, and the way it is situated in relation not only to my body but to my sense of myself. This is because proximities are always relational: in order to see substances and to see myself as being near or far, it is not enough to simply observe a material proximity constituted by the physical distances between things,

I also have to be able to judge the meanings of these distances. It is not only the fact that I am, right now, sitting in my apartment where my bathroom cabinet holds multiple opioid prescriptions that allows me to see myself as a "pain patient;" it is also the fact that I judge my proximity to these medications to be closer to the idea of a pain patient than to the idea of an addict, a drug abuser, a healthy person, and so forth. The imaginative dimensions of a material proximity serves to simultaneously construct a theoretical reality of a substance (that corresponds to its material reality) and *position me in relation to* this theoretical construction.

In doing so, this positioning is always a dialectical operation. My imaginative proximity to opioids creates my understanding of myself as a pain patient in part because it simultaneously constructs (and construes a personal distance from) the figure of an opioid addict, a figure farther away from my idea(l) of a pain patient; I can only judge something to be near when it is in relation to something else far away. And this operation is vital to understanding the importance and functioning of imaginative proximities within the opioid epidemic, because the theoretical — and social and linguistic — position of "I am a pain patient" corresponds to a material proximity and *maintains and reproduces the legal, biological, social, and personal consequences of this position.* "I am a pain patient" produces my legal ability to have multiple opioid prescriptions, my biological ability to experience the pain relief made possible by the continuation of this legal state, the fact that I can remain in a certain imaginative proximity to the future as predicated on these continuations, and so on. At the same time, how closely I am seen as truly and correctly in correspondence to others' idea(l)s of the position of a pain patient will not only contribute to these continued privileges, but will influence the treatment (or lack thereof) available for those seen as being far, as being opposite, from me.

The opioid epidemic is what is constructed around the opioid epidemic; the opioid epidemic is our collective (or cumulative) imaginative proximities to opioids. This is ultimately another way to name the affective structure of the epidemic: our imaginative proximities are what this epidemic feels like. And at no other time in the history of epidemiology has recognizing the importance of these theoretical relationships been as vital to creating an *after the epidemic*. The opioid epidemic is not an epidemic of a single disease, a single behavior, or even a single substance. Beyond the biological crisis and disease of addiction, the opioid epidemic *is* all of the sociopolitical, economic, and imaginative factors we have identified thus far. We will consistently fail in our efforts to address the physical experiences of addiction and pain until we fully recognize the influence of imaginative proximities in enabling abusive systemic distributions of opioids. Because, as placebo responses and speech acts teach us, when we shift our positions within theoretical relationships, we will alter the physical course of our own and others' bodies. When we decide and expect that we are about to experience pain relief, we do. When we decide and expect that methadone maintenance treatment is a positive experience and social good, the availability of which is about to produce huge positive changes in the course of the opioid epidemic, it will. When we decide that pain is just a substance like any other, that pain is something you can and will live with because "suffering is only *one* response to the experience of pain,"[28] and when we concurrently expect treatment options to become accessible and affordable and attendant to the social dimensions of pain, we will see huge positive change in the course of the opioid epidemic as opioid prescribing rates plummet. Even though, of course, these sequences of events are nowhere near as simple as these statements make them seem, it is also true that none of these things will happen until we first create these expectations of positivity around them. Because this has always been the story surrounding placebos, mind–body medicine, psychosomatic experiences — even exorcism, mesmerism, somnambulism — in that it was never only about a physical and psychological experience an individual was having, but the narratives and expectations that arose as many individuals repeatedly had those experiences. As these culturally specific and socially-circulating expectations and narratives drive governmental decision making, scientific research, and popular understandings over time, it becomes clear that what we expect

28 Jon Kabat-Zinn, *Full Catastrophe Living: Using the Wisdom of Your Body and Mind to Face Stress, Pain, and Illness* (New York: Penguin Random House, 1990), 285, emphasis in original.

to happen influences what does happen biologically as much as it does socially and politically. This is the essence of *expectation*: it is a form of cause and effect encapsulated in the wholeness of itself. Predicated as expectation is, etymologically, on the act of "looking out for," it becomes clear that we must decide what it is we are looking for only while recognizing that the ways we discuss and frame this, as well as the speech acts we therefore make possible, have and will continue to have profound physical effects — on all of us.

How can we begin to make these shifts in our imaginative proximities? In a way, these shifts must be functionally similar to the way in which addiction is approached through medical maintenance treatment: we must start by recognizing that taking away a substance does not alter or take away an underlying condition. That is, we cannot approach the goal of shifting our imaginative proximities in such a way that we implicitly attempt to only extricate ourselves, to become un-implicated and un-entangled from these relationships. Creating distances will not remove the two things that are in relation to each other. Instead, we can begin by recognizing that the constructed binaries created by the imaginative dimensions of our material proximities, of nearness/farness, pain patient/addict, use/abuse, are dialectics that can serve to create middle paths as much as to position two things as separate. Even distances that seem so far are relations that tie us together.

Under this fundamental condition — which is, in short, the impossibility of not being implicated — we can instead approach these shifts with the goal of creating imaginative proximities envisioned with "eyes of wholeness." In order to attend to our proximities to substances and to bodies always already deemed Other, we must first be able to shift our proximity to that deemed Normal — to an ideal, healthy, "substance-free" human body. Because without first recognizing and reorganizing our proximities to *a person, ourselves,* we will never be able to do so for others. Furthermore, without first recognizing the very specific form of wholeness underlying *a person, ourselves,* and the deeply problematic nature of the idea(l) of this wholeness, we will never be able to maintain proximities *with.*

The stakes in being able to achieve these are nothing less than the ability to find forms of freedom within the limitations of our proximities. Proximities that place us *with* — opioids, addiction, chronic illness, chronic pain — will only ever be oppressive within a rubric in which *wholeness, a person* only ever means a body *free from* everything: in which wholeness only ever means impenetrability, solidity, separation. But being *free from* is simply not the biological reality so many of us — the 2.1 million Americans with substance abuse issues, the 3,500 Americans who begin using opioids non-medicinally every day, the 100 million Americans living with chronic pain, every single person who will grow old and experience the infirmities of old age (and so on) — find ourselves within. We cannot continue asking how to be free from, how to *maintain* and *preserve* and *consume.* Instead: How do you live *with* something for a long time? How do you imagine yourself living with something for a long time? How do you recognize that, on a basic level, *with* is a metaphor that constructs companionship as much as it constructs instrumentality — that *with* is something you do, something you will use, as much as it is a way for understanding how that something feels?

All of these ideas — *imaginative proximity, living with, freedom with* — grew out of an idea that I became stuck on while reading about placebo responses and the opioid epidemic: the idea (creative or fantastical as it may be) that you could become addicted to thinking about your body in the future, in a different future. As if you could become addicted to the endorphins released in response to expectations of an *about to be* better body; as if I could sustain a fantasy like this for so long it would become a biological reality. But ultimately more interesting and pragmatic than the fascination this idea held for me is the reality of what are indeed relationships between illness, futurity, imagination, and co-constitutive realities therein. Somewhat tucked into the history of mind–body medicine and understandings of psychosomatic experiences is the history of post-traumatic stress disorder (PTSD). Whether it was called shell shock, battle fatigue, PTSD, or blast injuries, the physical and psychological trauma of war experiences has always existed. And within the diagnostic criteria for PTSD, there has long been a hallmark that became particularly striking within the context of the opioid epidemic and the endogenous and imaginative relations surrounding opioids: PTSD has long been characterized within the field of psychology by an inability to imagine a normal future, or an inability to imagine a return to normal life in the future. Given that the most recent research into PTSD, among Iraq War veterans, has found that it is often accompanied by very particular forms of scarring and injury within the brain — by very physical characteristics, that is — it is natural to assume that this situation demonstrates clear and direct links between a physical and psychological experience (being in a war; sustaining traumatic brain injuries through proximities to blasts and detonations) that augment one's imaginative proximity (here, to the idea of one's future) and that thereby produces further physical and psychological effects in perpetuity (the ongoing experience and symptoms of PTSD) with concurrent social and cultural effects seen in the meanings attributed to PTSD and the historically evolving nature of such meanings. Or, in other words, PTSD is a clear (if extreme) example of the way that trauma becomes diffuse and perpetuated through physical and imaginative experiences and relationships. Trauma and its movements through these zones of the psychosomatic, the psychological, the understood, the biological, is so much of what is folded into imaginative and material proximities. The trauma of pain and its chronicity, its material realities, shape my imaginative proximity to opioids — producing a theoretical relationship to them as *relief* — which in turn shapes my material and imaginative proximity to the future, through the expectations and ideas of *physical tolerance, ability, endurance.* The trauma of pain and precarity amid widespread economic recession shapes an imaginative proximity to the future — producing a theoretical relationship to futurity as *what will be possible?* — that in turn may shape a material proximity to opioids, understood within such an imaginative context as *pain relieving, sedating,* and which will, as we have continually seen, be a relationship of profound physical and imaginative effects projected far into the future. And this latter example, in particular, is far from hypothetical: as we have seen through examples, from time limits placed on opioid prescribing practices to the rise of neonatal abstinence syndrome, the relationship between physical trauma and futurity within the opioid epidemic is endemic and generational. As much as what is about to follow, here, may seem only theoretical or conceptual, I want to make clear that this trauma, pain, precarity, and the perpetuity of these states as imaginative and material realities is at the center of my thoughts. In thinking about freedom, about imaginative relationships, about creative understandings of biological realities, I am still never not thinking about the number of people dying in the time it is taking me to write this.

Freedom With

Freedom with is what arises when other forms of freedom become impossible. The material proximities so many of us — ultimately, all of us — are inhabiting within the opioid epidemic (as people with pain, as people with opioid addictions) have made certain forms of historically-valued freedom impossible. *Freedom with* arises in the impossibility of forms of freedom predicated, instead, on absences, removal, protection, wholeness-as-impenetrability, and other qualities emphasized in an atomistic and individualistic *freedom from*. *Freedom with* is what arises in the recognition of a state of *not aloneness,* a state of a molar individuality, of being a pack, a state of being sick forever, a state of being involved with or dependent on opioids forever, a state of being implicated forever, a state of *what is endogenous.* Detaching from the historically prioritized ideal of *freedom from,* a neoliberal ideal formulated as "freedom from encroachment by others and from collective institutions…[predicated on] an atomistic ontology, a metaphysics of separation, an ethos of defensiveness, and an abstract equality,"[29] means that *freedom with* need not be seen as (only) a failure to reach such ideals. In the absence of failure, one can instead approach these recognitions within a state closer to neutrality — an approach deeply rooted in the belief that "suffering is only *one* response."[30] An approach, that is, rooted in the belief that the way in which the opioid epidemic has figured the impossibility of *individuals free from* means that

29 Wendy Brown, *States of Injury: Power and Freedom in Late Modernity* (Princeton, NJ: Princeton University Press, 1995), 6.
30 Kabat-Zinn, *Full Catastrophe Living,* 285.

we must no longer continue attending to this situation only through attempts at returning to a conceptual status quo, to a collective imaginative proximity to an ideal of whole, normal, individuals, of wholeness-as-impenetrability. I will never be free from pain, nor is it likely I will ever be free from pain medications (or any of the other fifteen pills I take daily). This is not inherently negative. In the absence of being able to experience and rely on a sense of individuality as a sense of separateness, *freedom with* is the ability to find a form of freedom predicated on substance, porosity, interpenetration, circulations, flows of intensities, on what it feels like, on talking about what it feels like, on the things you do every day, on the things you have no choice but to do every day, on being able to say *because, with,* and *and,* and never only *in spite of.* Ultimately, this is a freedom based on the normality of our most visceral experiences and the fact that we are all, inextricably, together within them. *Freedom with* is the form of freedom possible within what is systemic and endogenous: everything, this.

In fact, the state of an endogenous substantiality is so fundamental to the concept of *freedom with* that it is not at all "posited independently of specific analyses of contemporary modalities of domination,"[31] as initial formulations of freedom frequently are. Instead, *freedom with* is so deeply tied to these contemporary modalities — to what is abusive and systemic — that *freedom with* is predicated on a biologically identical substance. *Freedom with* takes as one of its starting points that the endogenous nature of opioids is as much the meaning of *systemic* as the external, exogenous distribution of them. Particularly in this way, inasmuch as *freedom with* conceptually mirrors the physical flows and proximities and constantly fluctuating nature of opioids, *freedom with* is "a relational and contextual practice."[32] It is a state of freedom that is rickety, that folds and flows and exists always in part in the "increasingly subtle fluid" and "perceptual displacement of contours" that arises in relation between two things, between not always knowing where one thing ends and

---

31 Brown, *States of Injury,* 6.
32 Brown, *States of Injury,* 6.

the other begins.[33] There can be no separation from what is at the heart of this epidemic. How do you clearly identify the point at which the opioids already in your body, the endorphins, are truly any different from those circulating in anyone else's body? How much does the state of having been manufactured, of being exogenous, truly change the substantial nature of an opioid — is this not a change in form more than substance? And of what use is it, really, to look only for these differences? Who benefits from doing so? Nowhere within the opioid epidemic and within any imaginative proximity to it is a "metaphysics of separation" appropriate, as these practices would support.

This is not only because of the endogenous nature of opioids, but because of the way that ongoing situations perpetuate themselves in increasingly embedded ways that often remain imperceptible, at least to a certain point. At this moment, for example, there has been a significant rise in the number of organ donations made by those dying of drug overdoses; a rise that has gone relatively unnoticed. In 2016, there were 790 organ donations following overdose deaths, double the number seen in 2010. The 69 donations that occurred in New England alone represent transplants for 202 people.[34] A major factor driving this shift in donation trends is parallel to the epidemiology of the epidemic overall: deaths from traffic accidents have long been associated with organ donations (to the extent that organ donors are noted on driver's licenses), but overdose deaths surpassed those from traffic accidents in 2014; both are generally the sudden cause of death for younger, healthier people. It would be tempting, though difficult, to see within this situation some form of silver lining, if only because of the exponential way that organ donations benefit others (as multiple people can receive different organs from a single donor), but a more fundamental point to note is: the epidemic is having far-reaching effects that

33 Giles Deleuze, "The Fold," trans. Jonathan Strauss, *Yale French Studies* 80 (1991): 227–47, at 230, 246, https://doi.org/10.2307/2930269.
34 Katharine Q. Seelye, "As Drug Deaths Soar, a Silver Lining for Transplant Patients," *The New York Times,* October 6, 2016, https://www.nytimes.com/2016/10/06/us/as-drug-deaths-soar-a-silver-lining-for-organ-transplant-patients.html.

are bringing us closer and closer together — biologically as much as socially — in ways that we may not be able to fully recognize for years to come, but that we cannot ignore in the meantime.

Because of this interconnectedness and the relational forms yet to fully emerge, in combination with the impossibility of being *free from* that an experience and idea of *freedom with* represents, means that on a basic level, *freedom with* is a project of the decentralization of the individual; it is a project predicated on the building up of samenesses. In doing so, it inherently provides a counterpoint to the normative identity politics and categories underlying such politics — healthy, disabled, junkie, clean, abuse, dependent — whose existence (and, in cases like "white, rural, 23 years old," the dissolve of which) has fueled so many of the narratives, discriminatory politics, and pain within the epidemic. Detaching from these categories similarly means being able to detach from — to hope to avoid — a common paradox of freedom as freedom becomes institutionalized: "Institutionalized freedom [becomes] arrayed against a particular image of unfreedom [and] sustains that image, which dominates political life with its specter long after it has been vanquished."[35] That is, as "pain patient" is cemented further and further as the opposite of "addict," what becomes sustained is not only the freedoms of being a pain patient but the unfreedoms of being an addict. Despite the fact that doing so implies a failure to recognize the sameness of the biological realities at hand, that physical dependence and abuse lie along a gradient that is not only nowhere near as black and white as it may seem, but is also a gradient on which the substance at either end is identical. Recognizing a fundamental sameness means recognizing that there are no two sides to the epidemic, that we cannot be on different sides.

As what necessitates the ability to find forms of *freedom with* is the state of existing within relationships that, while plastic, are not endlessly flexible nor ever fully reversible — the state, in other words, of being people in pain and in addiction — it is not only the ideal of *freedom from* that has become impossible. Similarly, *freedom with* arises in the impossibility of achieving idealized forms of *freedom-as-mastery*. Opioids and pain, as substances

35 Brown, *States of Injury,* 8.

that are companions, that we are *with* — and that are therefore instrumental more in the sense of being substantial, important, and useful than they are simply tools to be wielded — means that these are not things over which we will ever be able to wield absolute power. Doing so would only be another iteration of a *freedom from*; in this case, a freedom from the "at the mercy of the body" narrative, a freedom from the body itself and even from the most basic biological functions of that body: pain and reward. There is no freedom possible within pain or addiction of *mind-from-body* or of *mind-over-body*. A Cartesian sense of mind–body separation is a privilege. Only those who have not yet been made viscerally aware of the forever and inherent concreteness of the "two" can continue to think of mind–body as such. For those of us who will instead, forever, say "being sick" and "being addicted," and never only "being," this privilege is an impossibility.

And it is at this point that it becomes important to acknowledge what may be a central criticism of the idea of a *freedom with*: the specter of biological determinism. It is not an easy criticism to answer, because the fact is that recognizing and stating a physical permanency to pain, to opioid addiction, and simultaneously tying this permanency to the imaginative, theoretical, freedom-effecting possibilities is, in fact, a form of biological determinism. The differences between these sentiments and the biological determinist attitudes coursing elsewhere in the epidemic are fine-grained but important. To recognize the fundamental reorganization of a life that happens, that must happen, in the event and cementing of pain or of addiction is not, in and of itself, to re-inscribe narratives of the standing of addicted or ill people as victims and perpetrators. Instead, it is really to theoretically prioritize the scene of the everyday, of what happens on a daily basis, on what these days feel like. It is not to say *once an addict, always an addict*; it is to say *this is what today feels as an addict and why tomorrow may feel similar.* "Daily" is not the same as "stagnant." A form of *freedom with* is still a form of freedom.

Furthermore, it may be tempting and easy to see, within the opioids that are endogenous, a scenario in which we all have the power to produce placebo responses within ourselves (and must therefore have the power to create limitless pain relief for ourselves) and, simultaneously, assume that this power is relative and determined within individuals by some kind of pre-existing criteria; criteria that may be variously called grit, resiliency, the power of a positive attitude, and so forth. On the contrary, it is exactly the relational, situational, engaged, and visceral aspects of the way that imaginative and material proximities influence an experience of *freedom with* that limits these assumptions. It is a form of freedom inherently not predetermined but shaped by current and ongoing experiences and proximities, and that responds to changes in these proximities as they happen.

There is a second criticism to note as well, one that could be leveled at any proposed conception of freedom. Initially, many such conceptions seem to cancel themselves out, a folding that occurs as: "Initial figurations of freedom are inevitably reactionary in the sense of emerging in reaction to perceived injuries or constraints of a regime from within its own terms. Ideals of freedom ordinarily emerge to vanquish their imagined immediate enemies, but in this move they frequently recycle and reinstate rather than transform the terms of domination that generated them."[36] However, it is exactly the importance of what is endogenous to this particular kind of *freedom with,* how what is endogenous is what allows such a formulation to emerge now, that is (at least an attempt to) avoid this conceptual operation. Built up from what is endogenous, made possible by the state of a substance within all of us that is one and the same as the substance of the opioid epidemic, there can be no attempt here to change the terms of what is happening, of what is actually causing and what is seen as causing current "perceived injuries or constraints." There is, instead, an attempt to reframe, to shift — to differently mobilize. To shift, that is, *opioids* as opioids are, stand for, and function as a substantial mixture of material, socioeconomic, political, and medical policies, narratives, and oppression enacted physically and taking place biologically. *Freedom with* and the endogenous situations motivating it recognizes this scene and works within exactly this place of the physical, the social, and personal, without attempting to change or remove or reverse it completely; because doing so would fly in

36 Brown, *States of Injury,* 7.

the face of the *impossibility of not being implicated* that a *freedom with* is predicated upon. Instead, by introducing into this mix and utilizing an imaginative proximity and recognizing the rippling influences of changes to this proximity, practices of *freedom with* within the epidemic can challenge and reverse the abusive flows we have seen throughout. One cannot immediately reverse the flow of opioids into and through the country, through our communities, and even, in many cases, through our own bodies, but with our expectations, our thoughts, our conversations, relations, and re-structuring of our affective scaffold, we can change *what is about to happen.* We can change the state of opioids, substantially; where they are about to be, where flows become eddies and where they become drifts.

In other words, we can, eventually, attempt to enter into and operate within "the organization of the activity through which the suffering is produced."[37] The opioid epidemic can only ever be fully addressed through opioids themselves, our proximities to them, and the policies these proximities and narratives engender. We cannot change the terms, the money, the history, or the deaths that opioids are, but we can shift the mixture of these systems within what opioids become. And what is so important to point out here, after this laying out of *freedom with,* and what must be held onto through these future attempts and our shifts within our own proximities, is that as much as it may seem that these terms (or their applications) are new here — or, while it may sound at the least unfamiliar and at the most fanciful or overly creative to consider the implications of endorphins and placebos within these terms — these ideas are not actually unfamiliar to many people, nor are they particularly new. As a pain patient and person working within the fields of critical theory and medical anthropology, I read Jon Kabat-Zinn as much as I read Foucault or Marx. I practice and attend to mindfulness, to the implications of dialectical behavioral therapy and cognitive therapy, to simply what is an actual experience of being in pain every day and probably forever, as much as I attend to conceptions of biopolitics, of Hegelian dialectics, of the history of medicine. Because of these scholarly, personal, and physical mixtures, the ideas of

37 Brown, *States of Injury,* 7.

freedom with and *imaginative proximity* and my understanding of placebo responses are, in a very real sense, a *Full Catastrophe Living* guide to living within an epidemic, or a critical theory version of *Full Catastrophe Living*. Given the enormous effect that Jon Kabat-Zinn's work has had on the fields of medical practice, psychology, and wellness in the United States, it is likely that these ideas and their applications are something that so many of us already know, have likely used ourselves, or have benefitted someone we know. Whether we would phrase it within these terms or not, many of us already understand imaginative proximities and their relations to material proximities to be a conduit for *living on,* for *living with.* The opioid epidemic is exactly what you know it to be. The opioid epidemic is exactly what you are already living.

The Opioid Epidemic: 1993-2017

Seeing with eyes of wholeness means recognizing that nothing occurs in isolation, that problems need to be seen within the context of whole systems. Seeing in this way, we can perceive the intrinsic web of interconnectedness underlying our experience and merge with it. Seeing in this way is healing.

— Jon Kabat-Zinn, *Full Catastrophe Living*[1]

The epidemic does not end in death. It is the way we live now, and we go on living.

— Jesse Erin Posner, private correspondence, 2017

The opioid epidemic is my lifetime. It is the lifetime, in fact, of all "Millennials," though especially those — younger, living in rural and suburban settings in extreme poverty — often left out of mainstream discussions of Millennials. How much of our lives will be filled with, by, opioids? My life? In what ways? How

[1]   Jon Kabat-Zinn, *Full Catastrophe Living: Using the Wisdom of Your Body and Mind to Face Stress, Pain, and Illness* (New York: Penguin Random House, 1990).

many opioid prescriptions will I fill in the next year? Ten years? What will my pain be like without them?

How many people, who I know, will die? How much time will I spend listening to people tell me about all of their friends who have died? How often will I be at my job, listening to a coworker tell a customer about her nephew's overdose death last summer? How often will I sit outside my house, listening to my neighbor tell me about all of the people from his hometown, on the North Shore of Massachusetts, who have died of opioid overdoses? How often will I be at work, listening to my coworker tell me about her partner's survived overdose? How often will I pass a local fast food restaurant and, seeing cop cars parked out front, immediately assume that there was an overdose in the public restroom there? How often will I pass people asleep on benches in Harvard Square, or nodding off on the bus, and worry that they've overdosed? Yesterday, I was walking to the grocery store and passed two men sitting on the front steps of a nearby apartment building. One of the men was leaning back, eyes closed, his mouth open and his arm, hand, outstretched. At what point did this become such an unmistakable posture? I wonder if this is a feature of heroin or of our thinking about heroin. What did we used to think?

It is a truly odd sensation to wish that one's writing is dated by the time it is published. But I do wish that I will have been wrong about a lot within the opioid epidemic. I wish that there would have been a series of public health, law enforcement, pain treatment, and addiction treatment breakthroughs; I wish that the opioid epidemic would have begun to get better by the end of 2017. However, especially given the ongoing dismantling of the US healthcare system and the repeated turning away from evidence-based addiction treatment, I do not think this will happen. In fact, according to a series of recent predictions developed by a varied group of epidemiologists and public health experts, the opioid epidemic will almost certainly get worse before it gets better. The worst of these predictions estimates 500,000 people dying in the United States over the next decade. This number is higher than deaths from AIDS *from the start of that epidemic* until now.[2]

The severity of this prediction may seem extreme, but has been mirrored by real-time events. In the spring of 2017, officials saw the appearance of carfentanil, the extremely potent synthetic opioid commonly used as an elephant tranquilizer, in Massachusetts for the first time.[3] This presence casts a sickening pall over the very idea of a public space. Who around you may be in possession of heroin tainted by carfentanil? How close are you to a substance that can be deadly to the touch, or to the inhalation? Is it not deeply disturbing that EMS responders are, or are considering, wearing HAZMAT suits when responding to overdoses? Whose body has become this dangerous? Whose pain is legal?

The kind of turning point marked by the appearance of carfentanil is not only an epidemic, law enforcement, and addiction-treatment turning point, but a personal one as well: I can't go on, with this, through this, much longer. If at all. I cannot continue to read constantly and solely about opioids, the deaths, the accidents, the failures of government, law enforcement, and medical bodies to respond effectively, the lack of other treatment options for managing pain. I cannot manage pain much longer, either, of any variety, without other options. I did not finish reading the article about the epidemic predictions, about the potential for 500,000 deaths. I simply cannot sustain this focus. Is it really so surprising that, after long-term intensive and immersive research in this situation, I have turned to topics like wellness, self-care, and the labor of illness for my next project?

But this doesn't mean, can't mean, that I can or want to stop paying attention altogether. I couldn't, even if I wanted

2   Max Blau, "STAT Forecast: Opioids Could Kill Nearly 500,000 Americans in the Next Decade," *STAT,* June 27, 2017, http://www. statnews.com/2017/06/27/opioid-deaths-forecast/.

3   Felicia Gans, "Three Samples of Carfentanil Found in Mass. for First Time," *The Boston Globe,* June 7, 2017, https://www.bostonglobe. com/metro/2017/06/07/state-police-find-three-traces-carfentanil-first-extremely-lethal-substance-found-massachusetts/qRJ9VqpoUc9feW-6zJawEoK/story.html.

to, because I still live here, still take painkillers, still listen to my friends and neighbors. I couldn't, even if I wanted to, because this has become the way we live now. And it is the way I live now. This project has always been motivated by the way I live now, by a sense — and lack thereof — of personal freedom. And this sense would have made it so easy to have written a book as a pain patient, or as a science journalist, or doctor, about the lack of adequate pain treatment, the history of anesthesia, or the detriments of the current opioid rhetoric on pain patients. But that would only ever have been a project and critique from the position of the injured, and I am always also implicated. Even as I am affected by the epidemic, do not always have nor may not continue to have access to adequate treatment, I am also deeply implicated in the broader systemic nature of the current situation. The mass of an epidemic is simply too large to allow for such simple and singular subject constructions: I am a pain patient and a patient without adequate pain treatment and a disabled person and a person who is going to be sick and a person who has given money to corporations involved in the manufacturing and marketing of opioids and a person who walks past people abusing drugs, probably opioids, without stopping and a person who could easily be addicted to these medications and a person whose taxes go, or don't go, to social services for addiction treatment, and on and on.

Which is what *freedom with* looks like, on a personal level. *Freedom with* takes place in all of these daily, and more than and less than daily, instances. Even recognizing and continually experiencing the difficulty in inhabiting these spaces, situations, and interstices between where one thing ends and another begins does not mean that I do not simultaneously recognize the value and importance of this kind of inhabitance. Being made of more than one thing is always better than being a single thing. I am not writing a self-help book; I don't think I need to provide specific suggestions, nor do I think that specific suggestions are always even possible to make. I think, instead, that the appropriate conclusion to an autoethnography of looking around is one that simply presents what has been seen.

This kind of shift, the change from continually reciting statistics about overdose rates, chronic pain epidemiology, and opioid prescribing rates to saying, instead, that this is the way we live now, is a very different kind of turning point than the one in which carfentanil appears in Massachusetts for the first time. This is the point at which, instead, the epidemic becomes something more than itself. Something more than any of the statistics or narratives or images can describe about it. The point at which it is recognized that the opioid epidemic is the way we live now is the point at which it has become, fully, my lifetime; our lifetimes.

And it was exactly this kind of experience that Susan Sontag illustrated in her 1986 short story "The Way We Live Now."[4] In it, a group of friends discusses an unnamed friend who is dying of AIDS. Other friends begin to get sick, to die, as well. AIDS shaped the lifetimes — was the lifetime — of a generation in much the same way that the opioid epidemic is (becoming) the lifetimes of many of us now. What is consistently amazing throughout their hospital visits, telephone conversations, and whispered remarks is the persistence of behaviors and attitudes — especially the petty, the quotidian, the jealous, but also the love and the friendship — through what is otherwise a horrific situation. The early years, especially, of the AIDS epidemic seem marked by exactly this kind of absorption of the catastrophic and horrific into the everyday. The persistence of the everyday through the epidemic and catastrophic is truly the point at which this is the way we live now.

As in, I'll continue to take my opioids as much as needed, even every day, because being able to do certain things (like cook and eat dinner with my family) is so valuable to me; it was the way I lived, and it is the way I live now. As in, I listen and attend on a daily basis to stories of pain, illness, and addiction, because these are my friends and neighbors; it was the way they lived, and it is the way we live now.

Some of these aspects, like any aspect of everyday life, will be choices that we have the privilege of making, and some will not. Some things we can choose to live with, some things we must simply move on through. Some things are an illness, some are

4   Susan Sontag, "The Way We Live Now," *The New Yorker,* November 24, 1986, https://www.newyorker.com/magazine/1986/11/24/the-way-we-live-now.

an epidemic. And epidemics that do not end become something altogether different.

But even in feeling despair or in being unable, consistently, to continue, I do not think this is a failure, a negative end point, or cause for a loss of hope. In concluding, I want to be deliberately inconclusive. Even as this is the way we live, it does not mean it is the way we will always live. What persists will be different.

BIBLIOGRAPHY

Acker, Caroline Jean. *Creating the American Junkie: Addiction Research in the Classic Era of Narcotic Control.* Baltimore, MD: Johns Hopkins University Press, 2002.

Achenbach, Joel, and Dan Keating. "A New Divide in American Death." *The Washington Post,* April 10, 2016. http://www. washingtonpost.com/sf/national/2016/04/10/a-new-divide-in-american-death/?utm_term=.3dbded6c06f5.

American Society of Addiction Medicine. "Opioid Addiction: 2016 Facts & Figures." n.d. http://www.asam.org/docs/default-source/advocacy/opioid-addiction-disease-facts-figures.pdf.

Annear, Steve. "Cambridge to Open City's First Freestanding Outdoor Public Toilet." *The Boston Globe,* February 8, 2016. https://www.bostonglobe.com/metro/2016/02/08/cambridge-open-city-first-freestanding-outdoor-public-toilet/WKAELRk7GpLPSUZg7xLCYI/story.html.

Anson, Pat. "Few Pain Patients Become Long-Term Opioid Users." *Pain News Network,* January 2, 2017. https://www.painnewsnetwork.org/stories/2017/1/2/few-pain-patients-become-long-term-opioid-users.

Armstrong, David. "Dope Sick." *STAT,* August 2, 2016. https://www.statnews.com/feature/opioid-crisis/dope-sick/.

Arnett, Jeffrey Jensen. *Emerging Adulthood: The Winding Road from the Late Teens through the Twenties.* Oxford: Oxford University Press, 2004.

Associated Press. "A Grim Tally Soars: More than 50,000 Overdose Deaths in US." *STAT,* December 9, 2016. https://www.statnews.com/2016/12/09/opoid-overdose-deaths-us/.

Associated Press and the Center for Public Integrity. "Drug Makers Push a Profitable but Unproven Opioid Solution." *STAT,* December 15, 2016. https://www.statnews.com/2016/12/15/drugmakers-unproven-opioid-solution/.

Austin, J.L. *How to Do Things with Words.* 2nd edn. Cambridge, MA: Harvard University Press, 1975.

Bebinger, Martha. "How Profits From Opium Shaped 19th-Century Boston." *CommonHealth* (blog), *WBUR,* July 31, 2017. http://www.wbur.org/commonhealth/2017/07/31/opium-boston-history.

———. "New Numbers Show Opioid Epidemic Rages on in Massachusetts." *CommonHealth* (blog), *WBUR,* August 3, 2016. http://www.wbur.org/commonhealth/2016/08/03/opioid-epidemic-numbers.

———. "Roughly 5 Mass. Residents Are Dying Daily Due to Overdose, Most Involving Fentanyl." *CommonHealth* (blog), *WBUR,* November 7, 2016. http://www.wbur.org/commonhealth/2016/11/07/overdose-deaths-fentanyl.

Benedetti, Fabrizio. "Drugs and Placebos: What's the Difference?" *EMBO Reports* 15, no. 4 (April 2014): 329–32. https://doi.org/10.1002/embr.201338399.

———, and Elisa Frisaldi. "Neurochemistry of Placebo Analgesia: Opioids, Cannabinoids and Cholecystokinin." In *Placebo and Pain: From Bench to Bedside,* eds. Luana Colloca, Magne Arve Flaten, and Karin Meissner, 9–14. London: Academic Press, 2013.

Benjamin, Walter. "The Work of Art in the Age of Mechanical Reproduction." In *Illuminations: Essays and Reflections,* ed. Hannah Arendt, trans. Harry Zohn, 217–52. New York: Schocken Books, 1968.

Berlant, Lauren. *Cruel Optimism.* Durham, NC: Duke University Press, 2011.

Blakemore, Paul R., and James D. White. "Morphine, the Proteus of Organic Molecules." *Chemical Communications* 11 (2002): 1159–68. https://doi.org/10.1039/B111551K.

Blau, Max. "STAT Forecast: Opioids Could Kill Nearly 500,000

Americans in the Next Decade." *STAT,* June 27, 2017. http://
www.statnews.com/2017/06/27/opioid-deaths-forecast/.

Borsook, David. "A Future Without Chronic Pain: Neuroscience
and Clinical Research." *Cerebrum: The Dana Forum on Brain
Science* (2012): 7. http://www.ncbi.nlm.nih.gov/pmc/articles/
PMC3574803/.

Bourgois, Philippe, and Jeffery Schonberg. *Righteous Dopefiend.*
Berkeley: University of California Press, 2009.

Bourke, Joanna. "This Won't Hurt a Bit: The Cultural
History of Pain." *New Statesmen,* June 19, 2014, 15–19.
https://www.newstatesman.com/culture/2014/06/
wont-hurt-bit-cultural-history-pain.

Brodwin, Erin. "A Searing New Report Claims Opioid
Drugmakers Spent 8 times as Much as the NRA on Lobbying."
Business Insider, September 19, 2016. http://www.
businessinsider.com/new-ap-report-opioid-drugmakers-
outspent-nra-lobbying-2016-9.

Brown, Wendy. *States of Injury: Power and Freedom in Late
Modernity.* Princeton, NJ: Princeton University Press, 1995.

Bruhm, Steven. *Gothic Bodies: The Politics of Pain in Romantic
Fiction.* Philadelphia: University of Pennsylvania Press, 1994.

Bureau of Justice Statistics. "Drugs and Crime Facts: Pretrial,
Prosecution and Adjudication." n.d. https://www.bjs.gov/
content/dcf/ptrpa.cfm.

Carson, Rachel. *Silent Spring.* Boston, MA: Houghton Mifflin,
1962.

Central Intelligence Agency (CIA). "The World Factbook: Illicit
Drugs." n.d. https://www.cia.gov/library/publications/the-
world-factbook/fields/2086.html.

Centers for Disease Control and Prevention (CDC). "Accidents or
Unintentional Injuries." Updated March 17, 2017. http://www.
cdc.gov/nchs/fastats/accidental-injury.htm.

———. "CDC Guideline for Prescribing Opioids for Chronic
Pain — United States, 2016." *Morbidity and Mortality
Weekly Report,* March 18, 2016. https://www.cdc.gov/mmwr/
volumes/65/rr/rr6501e1.htm.

———. "Opioid Overdose." 2016. https://www.cdc.gov/
drugoverdose/.

———. "Understanding the Epidemic." August 30, 2017. https://

www.cdc.gov/drugoverdose/epidemic/index.html.

Cherlin, Andrew J. "Why Are White Death Rates Rising?" *The New York Times,* February 22, 2016. http://www.nytimes.com/2016/02/22/opinion/why-are-white-death-rates-rising.html.

Cicero, Theodore J., Matthew S. Ellis, Hilary L. Surratt, et al. "The Changing Face of Heroin Use in the United States: A Retrospective Analysis of the Past 50 Years." *JAMA Psychiatry* 71, no. 7 (2014): 821–26. https://doi.org/10.1001/jamapsychiatry.2014.366.

Cohen, Jeff. "Details On Death Certificates Offer Layers Of Clues To Opioid Epidemic." *National Public Radio,* June 1, 2016. http://www.npr.org/sections/health-shots/2016/06/01/479440834/in-opioid-crisis-it-s-important-to-know-which-drugs-caused-a-death.

Colloca, Luana, and Fabrizio Benedetti. "Placebos and Painkillers: Is Mind as Real as Matter?" *Nature Reviews: Neuroscience* 6, no. 7 (July 2005): 545–52. https://doi.org/10.1038/nrn1705.

Corbett, Alistair D., Graeme Henderson, Alexander T. McKnight, and Stewart J. Paterson. "75 Years of Opioid Research: The Exciting but Vain Quest for the Holy Grail." *British Journal of Pharmacology* 147, no. S1 (2006): S153–S162. https://doi.org/10.1038/sj.bjp.0706435.

Courtwright, David T. *Forces of Habit: Drugs and the Making of the Modern World.* Cambridge, MA: Harvard University Press, 2002.

Damasio, Antonio. *The Feeling of What Happens: Body and Emotion in the Making of Consciousness.* New York: Harcourt Brace, 1999.

Davenport-Hines, Richard. *The Pursuit of Oblivion: A Global History of Narcotics.* New York: W.W. Norton, 2004.

Deleuze, Gilles. "The Fold," trans. Jonathan Strauss. *Yale French Studies* 80 (1991): 227–47. https://doi.org/10.2307/2930269.

———, and Félix Guattari. *A Thousand Plateaus: Capitalism and Schizophrenia,* trans. Brian Massumi. London: The Athlone Press, 1988.

Deyo, Richard A., Michael Von Korff, and David Duhrkoop. "Opioids for Low Back Pain." *British Medical Journal* 350 (2015): g6380. https://doi.org/10.1136/bmj.g6380.

Donnelly, Grace. "As Drug Overdoses Hit Record High, Trump
    Offers Little on Opioid Policy." *Fortune,* August 8, 2017. http://
    fortune.com/2017/08/08/record-high-drug-related-death-
    rate-2016/.

Drug Enforcement Agency (DEA). "DEA Report: Counterfeit Pills
    Fueling U.S. Fentanyl and Opioid Crisis." July 22, 2016. https://
    www.dea.gov/divisions/hq/2016/hq072216.shtml.

———. "Fentanyl." December 2016. https://www.deadiversion.
    usdoj.gov/drug_chem_info/fentanyl.pdf.

Ettlinger, Nancy. "Precarity Unbound." *Alternatives: Global,
    Local, Political* 32, no. 3 (2007): 319–40. https://doi.
    org/10.1177/030437540703200303.

Fine, Perry G. "Long-Term Consequences of Chronic Pain:
    Mounting Evidence for Pain as a Neurological Disease
    and Parallels with Other Chronic Disease States." *Pain
    Medicine* 12, no. 7 (July 2011): 996–1004. https://doi.
    org/10.1111/j.1526-4637.2011.01187.x.

Foreman, Judy. *A Nation in Pain: Healing Our Biggest Health
    Problem.* Oxford: Oxford University Press, 2014.

France, David, dir. *How to Survive a Plague.* New York: Public
    Square Films, 2012.

Franco, Celinda. "Drug Courts: Background, Effectiveness, and
    Policy Issues for Congress." Washington, DC: Congressional
    Research Service, 2010. https://fas.org/sgp/crs/misc/R41448.
    pdf.

Freyer, Felice J. "Overdose Deaths in Mass. Continue to
    Surge." *The Boston Globe,* November 7, 2016. https://www.
    bostonglobe.com/metro/2016/11/07/overdose-deaths-mass-
    continue-surge/z9AdKhXF43NAhngHYvTguO/story.html.

Frontline. *Chasing Heroin.* Arlington, VA: Public Broadcasting
    Service, 2016. https://www.pbs.org/wgbh/frontline/film/
    chasing-heroin/.

Gans, Felicia. "Three Samples of Carfentanil Found in Mass. for
    First Time." *The Boston Globe,* June 7, 2017. https://www.
    bostonglobe.com/metro/2017/06/07/state-police-find-three-
    traces-carfentanil-first-extremely-lethal-substance-found-
    massachusetts/qRJ9VqpoUc9feW6zJawEoK/story.html.

Gawande, Atul. *Being Mortal: Medicine and What Matters in the
    End.* New York: Metropolitan Books, 2014.

Gelburd, Robin. "The opioid epidemic is skyrocketing private insurance costs." *STAT,* September 26, 2016. https://www.statnews.com/2016/09/26/opioid-epidemic-private-insurance-payments/.

Glazek, Christopher. "The Secretive Family Making Billions From The Opioid Crisis." *Esquire,* October 16, 2017. https://www.esquire.com/news-politics/a12775932/sackler-family-oxycontin/.

Goldman, Bruce. "Study Reveals Brain Mechanism Behind Chronic Pain's Sapping of Motivation." *Stanford University Medicine News Center,* July 31, 2014. https://med.stanford.edu/news/all-news/2014/07/study-reveals-brain-mechanism-behind-chronic-pains-sapping-of-mo.html.

Goodnough, Abby. "Finding Good Pain Treatment is Hard. If You're Not White, It's Even Harder." *The New York Times,* August 10, 2016. http://www.nytimes.com/2016/08/10/us/how-race-plays-a-role-in-patients-pain-treatment.html.

Gura, Trisha. "When Pretending is the Remedy." *Scientific American Mind* 24, no. 1 (March/April 2013): 34–9.

Harrington, Anne. *The Cure Within: A History of Mind–Body Medicine.* New York: W.W. Norton, 2008.

Harvard T.H. Chan School of Public Health. "An Opioid Emergency." November 2, 2017. https://www.hsph.harvard.edu/news/multimedia-article/president-trump-opioid-emergency/.

Harvey, David. *A Companion to Marx's Capital.* New York: Verso, 2010.

Health and Human Services (HHS). "The Opioid Epidemic: By the Numbers." Updated January 2018. https://www.hhs.gov/opioids/sites/default/files/2018-01/opioids-infographic.pdf.

Healy, Maura. "Cutting Off the Opioid Epidemic at the Root." *The Boston Globe,* February 16, 2016. https://www.bostonglobe.com/opinion/2016/02/16/cutting-off-opioid-epidemic-root/EdovYeSsn5QbWtLY3ICY5J/story.html.

Heilig, Markus. *The Thirteenth Step: Addiction in the Age of Brain Science.* New York: Columbia University Press, 2015.

Howell, Tom, Jr. "Opioid Epidemic Demands Greater Access to Key Medications: Govt. Report." *The Washington Times,* October 27, 2016. http://www.washingtontimes.com/

news/2016/oct/27/opioid-epidemic-demands-access-key-meds-report.

Kabat-Zinn, Jon. *Full Catastrophe Living: Using the Wisdom of Your Body and Mind to Face Stress, Pain, and Illness.* New York: Penguin Random House, 1990.

Keane, Helen. "Public and Private Practices: Addiction Autobiography and its Contradictions." *Contemporary Drug Problems* 28, no. 4 (2001): 567–95. https://doi.org/10.1177/009145090102800404.

———. "Smoking, Addiction, and the Making of Time." In *High Anxieties: Cultural Studies in Addiction,* eds. Janet Farrell Brodie and Marc Redfield, 119–33. Berkeley: University of California Press, 2002.

———, and Kelly Hamill. "Variations in Addiction: The Molecular and the Molar in Neuroscience and Pain Medicine." *BioSocieties* 5, no. 1 (March 2010): 52–69. https://doi.org/10.1057/biosoc.2009.4.

Keefe, Patrick Radden. "The Family that Built an Empire of Pain." *The New Yorker,* October 30, 2017. https://www.newyorker.com/magazine/2017/10/30/the-family-that-built-an-empire-of-pain.

Kertesz, Stefan, and Sally Satel. "Some People Still Need Opioids." *Slate,* August 17, 2017. http://www.slate.com/articles/health_and_science/medical_examiner/2017/08/cutting_down_on_opioids_has_made_life_miserable_for_chronic_pain_patients.html.

Kraus, Lewis. "2016 Disability Statistics Annual Report." Durham, NH: University of New Hampshire, 2017. https://disabilitycompendium.org/sites/default/files/user-uploads/2016_AnnualReport.pdf.

Lakoff, George, and Mark Johnson. *Metaphors We Live By.* Chicago: University of Chicago Press, 1980.

Leslie, Ian. "The Sugar Conspiracy." *The Guardian,* April 7, 2016. https://www.theguardian.com/society/2016/apr/07/the-sugar-conspiracy-robert-lustig-john-yudkin.

Ludden, Jennifer. "An Even Deadlier Opioid, Carfentanil, is Hitting the Streets." *National Public Radio,* September 2, 2016. http://www.npr.org/sections/health-shots/2016/09/02/492108992/

an-even-deadlier-opioid-carfentanil-is-hitting-the-streets.

Marchant, Jo. *Cure: A Journey into the Science of Mind Over Body.* New York: Crown, 2016.

———. "Strong Placebo Response Thwarts Painkiller Trials." *Nature News,* October 6, 2015. http://www.nature.com/news/strong-placebo-response-thwarts-painkiller-trials-1.18511.

———. "You Can Train Your Body into Thinking It's Had Medicine." *Mosaic,* Feb. 9, 2016. https://mosaicscience.com/story/medicine-without-the-medicine-how-to-train-your-immune-system-placebo.

Massachusetts Department of Public Health. "Data Brief: An Assessment of Opioid-Related Deaths in Massachusetts, 2013–2014." September 2016. https://www.mass.gov/files/documents/2017/08/31/chapter-55-opioid-overdose-study-data-brief-9-15-2016.pdf.

———. "Data Brief: Opioid-related Overdose Deaths Among Massachusetts Residents." August 2016. http://www.mass.gov/eohhs/docs/dph/quality/drugcontrol/county-level-pmp/opioid-related-overdose-deaths-among-ma-residents-august-2016.pdf.

———. "Number of Unintentional Opioid-Related Overdose Deaths by County, MA Residents: 2000–2015." November 2016. http://www.mass.gov/eohhs/docs/dph/stop-addiction/current-statistics/overdose-deaths-by-county-nov-2016.pdf.

Massachusetts Judicial Branch. "Drug Courts: Facts and Statistics." 2016. http://www.mass.gov/courts/programs/specialty-courts/drug-courts-facts-and-statistics.html.

McCoy, Alfred. "From Free Trade to Prohibition: A Critical History of the Modern Asian Opium Trade." *Fordham Urban Law Journal* 28, no. 1 (2000): 307–49. https://ir.lawnet.fordham.edu/ulj/vol28/iss1/4/.

Meek, Allen. *Biopolitical Media: Catastrophe, Immunity and Bare Life.* New York: Routledge, 2016.

Meldrum, Marcia L. "A Capsule History of Pain Management." *Journal of the American Medical Association* 290, no. 18 (2003): 2470–75. https://doi.org/10.1001/jama.290.18.2470.

Mettler, Katie. "'This is unprecedented': 174 Heroin Overdoses in 6 Days in Cincinnati." *Chicago Tribune,* August 29, 2016. http://www.chicagotribune.com/news/nationworld/midwest/

ct-heroin-overdose-outbreak-20160829-story.html.

Mold, Alex. "Consuming Habits: Histories of Drugs in Modern Societies." *Culture and Social History* 4, no. 2 (2007): 261–70. https://doi.org/10.2752/147800307X199074.

Morell, Alex. "The OxyContin Clan: The $14 Billion Newcomer to Forbes 2015 List of Richest U.S. Families." *Forbes,* July 1, 2015. http://www.forbes.com/sites/alexmorrell/2015/07/01/the-oxycontin-clan-the-14-billion-newcomer-to-forbes-2015-list-of-richest-u-s-families/#14cb7821c0e2.

Motluck, Alison. "Placebos Trigger an Opioid Hit in the Brain." *The New Scientist,* August 23, 2015. https://www.newscientist.com/article/dn7892-placebos-trigger-an-opioid-hit-in-the-brain/.

NAACP. "Criminal Justice Fact Sheet." n.d. http://www.naacp.org/pages/criminal-justice-fact-sheet.

National Institute of Justice. "Drug Courts." January 10, 2017. http://www.nij.gov/topics/courts/drug-courts/pages/welcome.aspx.

National Institute on Drug Abuse (NIDA). "Increased Drug Availability is Associated with Increased Use and Overdose." January 2018. https://www.drugabuse.gov/publications/research-reports/relationship-between-prescription-drug-abuse-heroin-use/increased-drug-availability-associated-increased-use-overdose.

National Institutes of Health Pain Consortium. "Disparities in Pain Care." n.d. https://www.ninds.nih.gov/sites/default/files/DisparitiesPainCare.pdf.

Nolan, Dan, and Chris Amico. "How Bad is the Opioid Epidemic?" *PBS Frontline,* February 23, 2016. http://www.pbs.org/wgbh/frontline/article/how-bad-is-the-opioid-epidemic/.

Northwestern University News. "Chronic Pain Shrinks 'Thinking Parts' Of Brain." November 23, 2004. http://www.northwestern.edu/newscenter/stories/2004/11/chronic.html.

Pizzo, Philip A., and Noreen M. Clark. "Alleviating Suffering 101 — Pain Relief in the United States." *New England Journal of Medicine* 366, no. 3 (January 2012): 197–99. https://doi.org/10.1056/NEJMp1109084.

Quinones, Sam. *Dreamland: The True Tale of America's Opiate Epidemic.* London: Bloomsbury, 2015.

Ramos, Nestor, and Evan Allan. "Life and Loss on Methadone Mile." *The Boston Globe,* July 2016. https://apps.bostonglobe.com/graphics/2016/07/methadone-mile/.

Rodriguez-Raecke, Rea, Andreas Niemeier, Kristin Ihle, Wolfgang Reuther, and Arne May. "Brain Gray Matter Decrease in Chronic Pain is the Consquence and Not the Cause of Pain." *Journal of Neuroscience* 29, no. 44 (November 2009): 13746–50. https://doi.org/ 10.1523/JNEUROSCI.3687-09.2009.

Rudd, Rose A., Puja Seth, Felicita David, and Lawrence Scholl. "Increases in Drug and Opioid-Involved Overdose Deaths–United States, 2010–2015." *Morbidity and Mortality Weekly Report.* Centers for Disease Control and Prevention (CDC), December 30, 2016. https://www.cdc.gov/mmwr/volumes/65/wr/mm6550e1.htm.

Saslow, Eli. "How's Amanda? A Story of Truth, Lies, and an American Addiction." *The Washington Post,* July 23, 2016. http://www.washingtonpost.com/sf/national/2016/07/23/numb/.

Saunders, Cicely. "Into the Valley of the Shadow of Death: A Personal Therapeutic Journey." *British Medical Journal* 313, no. 7072 (December 1996): 1599–1601. http://hdl.handle.net/10822/898833.

Scarry, Elaine. *The Body in Pain: The Making and Unmaking of the World.* Oxford: Oxford University Press, 1985.

Schofferman, Jerome, Scott M. Fishman, and R. Norman Harden. "Did We Reach Too Far? The Opioid Epidemic and Chronic Pain." *American Academy of Physical Medicine and Rehabilitation* 6, no. 1 (Januray 2014): 78–84. https://doi.org/10.1016/j.pmrj.2013.12.003.

Scott, Dylan. "1 in 3 Americans Blame Doctors for National Opioid Epidemic, STAT-Harvard Poll Finds." *STAT,* March 17, 2016. https://www.statnews.com/2016/03/17/stat-harvard-opioid-poll/.

Seelye, Katharine Q. "As Drug Deaths Soar, a Silver Lining for Transplant Patients." *The New York Times,* October 6, 2016. https://www.nytimes.com/2016/10/06/us/as-drug-deaths-soar-a-silver-lining-for-organ-transplant-patients.html?ref=todayspaper&_r=0.

———. "Heroin Epidemic Increasingly Seeps Into Public View."

The New York Times, March 7, 2016. https://www.nytimes.
com/2016/03/07/us/heroin-epidemic-increasingly-seeps-into-
public-view.html.

Silberman, Steve. "Placebos Are Getting More Effective: Drug
Makers Are Desperate to Know Why." *WIRED,* August 24,
2009. https://www.wired.com/2009/08/ff-placebo-effect/.

Sherman, Jennifer. "Rural Poverty: The Great Recession, Rising
Unemployment and the Under-utilized Safety Net." In *Rural
America in a Globalizing World Problems and Prospects for the
2010s,* eds. Conner Bailey, Leif Jensen, and Elizabeth Ransom,
523–42. Morgantown: West Virginia University Press, 2014.

Sontag, Susan. *Illness as Metaphor and AIDS and its Metaphors.*
New York: Farrar, Straus and Giroux, 1978.

———. "The Way We Live Now." *The New Yorker,* November
24, 1986. https://www.newyorker.com/magazine/1986/11/24/
the-way-we-live-now.

Struthers, Cynthia B. "The Past is the Present: Gender and the
Status of Rural Women." In *Rural America in a Globalizing
World Problems and Prospects for the 2010s,* eds. Conner Bailey,
Leif Jensen, and Elizabeth Ransom, 489–505. Morgantown:
West Virginia University Press, 2014.

Szalavitz, Maia. "How America Overdosed on Drug Courts."
Pacific Standard Magazine, May 18, 2005. https://psmag.com/
how-america-overdosed-on-drug-courts.

Tedeschi, Bob. "A 'Civil War' Over Painkillers Rips Apart the
Medical Community — and Leaves Patients in Fear." *STAT,*
January 17, 2017. https://www.statnews.com/2017/01/17/
chronic-pain-management-opioids/

US Department of Justice, Drug Enforcement Administration.
"Fentanyl: A Briefing Guide for First Responders."
June 2017. https://www.dea.gov/druginfo/Fentanyl_
BriefingGuideforFirstResponders_June2017.pdf.

Volkow, Nora D. "America's Addiction to Opioids: Heroin
and Prescription Drug Abuse." National Institute on Drug
Abuse (NIDA), May 14, 2014. https://www.drugabuse.gov/
about-nida/legislative-activities/testimony-to-congress/2018/
americas-addiction-to-opioids-heroin-prescription-drug-abuse.

———. "What Science Tells Us About Opioid Abuse and
Addiction." National Institute on Drug Abuse (NIDA),

January 27, 2016. https://www.drugabuse.gov/about-nida/legislative-activities/testimony-to-congress/2018/what-science-tells-us-about-opioid-abuse-addiction.

Wapner, Jessica. "Austin, Indiana: The HIV Capital of Small-town America." *Mosaic,* May 2, 2016. https://mosaicscience.com/story/austin-indiana-hiv-america-syndemics.

"The local mechanisms of mind . . . are not all in the head.

Cognition leaks out into body and world."

— Andy Clark, *Supersizing the Mind*

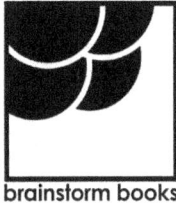
brainstorm books

Current developments in psychoanalysis, psychology, philosophy, and cognitive and neuroscience confirm the profound importance of expression and interpretation in forming the mind's re-workings of its intersubjective, historical and planetary environments. Brainstorm Books seeks to publish cross-disciplinary work on the becomings of the extended and enactivist mind, especially as afforded by semiotic experience. Attending to the centrality of expression and impression to living process and to the ecologically-embedded situatedness of mind is at the heart of our enterprise. We seek to cultivate and curate writing that attends to the ways in which art and aesthetics are bound to, and enhance, our bodily, affective, cognitive, developmental, intersubjective, and transpersonal practices.

Brainstorm Books is an imprint of the "Literature and the Mind" group at the University of California, Santa Barbara, a research and teaching concentration hosted within the Department of English and supported by affiliated faculty in Comparative Literature, Religious Studies, History, the Life Sciences, Psychology, Cognitive Science, and the Arts.

http://mind.english.ucsb.edu/brainstorm-books/

Brainstorm Books

www.ingramcontent.com/pod-product-compliance
Lightning Source LLC
Chambersburg PA
CBHW050651270326
41927CB00012B/2983